# THE REPRODUCTION OF INEQUALITY

HEALTH, SOCIETY, AND INEQUALITY SERIES
General Editor: Jennifer A. Reich

*Elder Care in Crisis: How the Social Safety Net Fails Families*
Emily K. Abel

*The Reproduction of Inequality: How Class Shapes the Pregnant Body and Infant Health*
Katherine Mason

# The Reproduction of Inequality

*How Class Shapes the Pregnant Body
and Infant Health*

Katherine Mason

**NEW YORK UNIVERSITY PRESS**
New York

NEW YORK UNIVERSITY PRESS
New York
www.nyupress.org

© 2023 by New York University
All rights reserved

Please contact the Library of Congress for Cataloging-in-Publication data.
ISBN: 9781479801954 (hardback)
ISBN: 9781479801947 (paperback)
ISBN: 9781479801909 (library ebook)
ISBN: 9781479801916 (consumer ebook)

New York University Press books are printed on acid-free paper, and their binding materials are chosen for strength and durability. We strive to use environmentally responsible suppliers and materials to the greatest extent possible in publishing our books.

Manufactured in the United States of America

10 9 8 7 6 5 4 3 2 1

Also available as an ebook

*For Jamie, whose bodily joy is breathtaking beyond measure.*

# CONTENTS

# Introduction

I met thirty-two-year-old Stephanie Brewer on a rainy December morning at a small, independent coffee shop in California's San Francisco Bay Area. A tall, youthful-looking white woman with a high ponytail and brightly colored rain boots, Stephanie had two young children: four-year-old Olive and one-and-a-half-year-old Felix. Stephanie had a husband who earned a six-figure salary and a graduate degree herself, but she had scaled back from full-time work while her children were little. Sipping a steaming mug of coffee, Stephanie recalled the health resolutions she had made during her first pregnancy five years before: "With Olive, I wanted to have the absolute perfect pregnancy, because I wanted her to have the best start in life. And so it was like, 'Okay, I need to eat fish twice a week. I need to eat this and that. . . .' I've always had a diet that's very low in processed foods, I've always had a diet that's very low in junk. I've never been an empty calorie person. But I was much more aware of what I was eating, because I was eating for a purpose."

Among the seventy women I interviewed for this book, nearly all voiced a similar sentiment: regardless of previous health or lifestyle habits, pregnancy was a time for examining and adjusting those habits in order to have a healthy baby. Over the course of 2010–2011, I spoke to women from multiple US states, diverse racial/ethnic groups, and an array of socioeconomic statuses about their body-care practices during this period.[1] My goal was to understand the external and internalized pressures on mothers to be healthy—as well as what "health" meant to each woman—during pregnancy and in the months and years following it. Furthermore, I wondered how those pressures (or women's responses to them) might shape or be shaped by social status.

Stephanie's hopes for giving Olive the "best start in life" did not end with pregnancy. After giving birth, she resolved to breastfeed Olive for at least a year. Her body, however, had other plans:

With Olive, I was like, "Well, I'm breastfeeding. I'm going to do it for a year. That's what the AAP [American Academy of Pediatrics] says, I'm going to do it for a year." So I was devastated when I dried up at nine months and she just weaned overnight. We had been doing some formula to supplement, because my supply was going down, and Olive didn't miss a beat. But I was so upset. Because I was supposed to go a whole year. I *wanted* to go a whole year, and I wasn't ready to be done. It took me probably a year to realize that she wasn't at a detriment because of what happened. Our relationship wasn't impacted, her health wasn't impacted, her development wasn't impacted. But there is this information overload [that new moms get] that says, "Breastfeed for X, Y, Z reasons."

At the time Olive was born, the AAP's "breast is best" approach recommended exclusive breastfeeding (human milk, not commercial infant formula, as a baby's only food) during the first six months of an infant's life, with mothers continuing to offer breastmilk alongside solid foods until at least the child's first birthday.[2] Medical authorities touted this practice as beneficial for children's health and development and for mother-child bonding. Like most middle- and upper-class mothers I interviewed, Stephanie was familiar with these recommendations and made a plan to follow them. Stephanie explained to me that when she was unable to stick to the plan—when her body's milk supply diminished beyond her control—she felt that she had failed as a mother.

A few weeks later, and about thirty miles inland, I met Gaby Romero at her home. Gaby was a first-generation Honduran immigrant who, at the age of twenty-nine, had given birth to her first child a month earlier. Still in maternity clothes and wearing her curly hair pulled back, Gaby cradled her sleeping infant and described her transition into motherhood. Gaby's pregnancy had not been easy—she had gained almost sixty pounds and was diagnosed with gestational diabetes, for which her doctors prescribed a restrictive diet—and Gaby worried about the health consequences her son might face: "I was surprised to have [gestational diabetes]. And then a lot of the girls who were going through it were saying 'Oh, when the baby's born it's going to go away,' but I was freaking out because my grandma died, and she had diabetes, and my aunt died too and had diabetes too, and my dad has it. I was like, 'Wow, the baby's going to have it.' So I was like, 'I really need to find some resources. I need to find out about good eating habits.'"

Gaby's doctor referred her to the Women, Infants, and Children (WIC) program, a federal program that provides free food and nutritional counseling to low-income women and children under five. Despite WIC's wide reach—more than 50 percent of US children receive WIC aid at some point in their first five years of life—Gaby, who was married and worked as a medical assistant, was surprised to learn that she qualified.[3] She initially had reservations about accepting what she viewed as a government handout, but she came to appreciate the nutritional information WIC provided, explaining, "I'm a picky eater, and I don't really like to eat a lot of fruit and stuff, but since I've been in the program because of the baby, I've been changing my habits of eating. And that's a good benefit for me and for the baby."

Like Stephanie, Gaby saw pregnancy as a time to make changes to her health practices for the sake of the child she was expecting. Unlike Stephanie, who aimed to improve on her already-meticulous eating practices in order to have the "absolute perfect pregnancy," Gaby focused on addressing nutritional deficits to protect her child from the diabetes and early mortality that ran in her family. Changing her eating habits meant swapping out familiar fare like tortillas (she did not like the whole wheat ones WIC provided) in favor of foods like celery sticks with peanut butter, which she disliked but ate for her son's sake. After her son was born, Gaby continued to follow WIC's advice by initiating breastfeeding.

I remember going to the breastfeeding class and their number one issue is advising you to breastfeed. [The counselor's] like, "Make a goal for at least six weeks or six months, but the best is for a year." And I got that into my mentality: "You know what? I want to breastfeed. I really don't want my baby to try anything but my breastmilk, just because of all the benefits from the breastmilk." I remember talking to the lactation counselor and I told her after the baby was born, "Oh my god, he's so used to it. I don't think I can do this anymore. It's taking all my energy. He's on my breast all the time, and that's the only thing he eats." And she's like, "Yeah, you did a good job, you need to continue doing it." I'm like, "I only want to do it for a small amount," but she's like, "No, you're doing great." So, they encourage you so much to breastfeed the kid, and I think it's good. . . . but then at the same time, I'm like, "What did I get myself into?" Now he doesn't want to do the formula or the bottle. . . . His body's so much for me. And when I go back to work it's going to be hard for both of us.

Gaby, like Stephanie, was convinced of the benefits of breastmilk, and she planned to exclusively breastfeed when her son was born. Nevertheless, as the weeks went on, she was exhausted by the hours she spent feeding her son each day, and she worried about how her bottle-averse child would fare when she had to return to work in a few weeks. Many other low-income women I spoke to voiced related concerns: for some, breastfeeding was a painful ordeal that they endured as long as they could before switching to formula; others felt uncomfortable or self-conscious about the bodily act of breastfeeding, particularly when they belonged to communities where breastfeeding was uncommon; and still others worried that their babies were not getting enough nourishment from their milk. WIC staff members tried to reassure these women and encourage them to keep going, but Gaby and others questioned whether the potential, uncertain benefits of extended breastfeeding might be out-weighed by other, more tangible benefits: holding down a full-time job, returning to school, and sharing feeding and caregiving responsibilities with a partner or other family members.

Gaby and Stephanie encountered similar bodily experiences and challenges on the road to motherhood, and both made choices about caring for their bodies in light of mainstream health guidelines. Yet their health practices—and their feelings about those practices—often differed quite drastically. Specifically, Stephanie approached the bodily demands of new motherhood with excitement, enthusiastically pursuing what she believed to be an optimal pregnancy diet and investing herself in a plan to breastfeed for the first year, so much so that she mourned the premature end of lactation. Gaby's feelings were decidedly mixed. Like Stephanie, she made dietary changes during pregnancy and followed advice to exclusively breastfeed her child, believing these practices would benefit her son. Unlike Stephanie, she did so ambivalently: many of the foods she was told to eat were distasteful to her, and she found breastfeeding both physically uncomfortable and time-consuming.

The differences in how Stephanie and Gaby approached the work of caring for their maternal bodies reflect, in a number of ways, broader trends I observed across classes: middle- and upper-class women like Stephanie tended to pour all of their energies into optimizing pregnancy and breastfeeding outcomes, enthusiastically describing their health choices and detailing the decision-making processes leading up to those choices; poor and working-class women like Gaby, on the other hand, focused more on mitigating harm and strategically investing, making lifestyle changes at times they perceived would yield the greatest benefits and framing those efforts as self-sacrifice, not self-expression. And while middle- and upper-class mothers emphasized the lengths to which they would go to avoid future risks—implying that no cost was too great when it came to their children's health and development—poor and working-class women directed their time and energy toward immediate health issues while questioning the value of practices aimed at avoiding hypothetical future risks.

*The Reproduction of Inequality* asks, What accounts for these class differences in pregnancy and postpartum body-care practices, and what might be the effects for mothers and children? One set of contributors is *economic*. Middle- and upper-class women tend to have more disposable income to spend on special health products and services; high-quality private health insurance; and jobs with flexible work schedules and comparatively generous parental leave benefits. Poor and working-class women, meanwhile, are more likely to use low-cost or publicly subsidized health services; to have minimal or no health insurance coverage; and to work in low-wage jobs with little flexibility or paid maternity leave. As later chapters will explore, these material differences between women across classes made a real difference in their ability to select and consume the health-related goods and services that fit their needs. A second possible contributor to these patterns of health behavior is class differences in health literacy and body-care *information*. By design, middle- and upper-class women in my study had higher levels of formal education—a bachelor's degree or higher—than those in the poor and working-class group. Such disparities could potentially lead to differences in, for example, scientific knowledge (through academic coursework or career expertise) or critical-reading skills for researching and interpreting medical guidance. Higher- and lower-class women belong to different social networks, and those networks tend to be class and racially segregated; thus, the informal knowledges about health that they access through peers and family members are different, too. Aid programs like WIC have long claimed that low-income women and children are less healthy because they lack accurate information about nutrition. Attempting to remedy this, WIC requires participants to attend nutrition workshops and receive one-on-one counseling as a condition of receiving financial assistance.

Both of these factors—financial status and health literacy—give us part of the picture. But both offer fundamentally *deficit-based* explanations for class differences in health or health practices: middle- and upper-class women's bodies and habits are typically treated as the norm, and poor and working-class women's approaches are defined by what they lack. Yet, financial and informational privilege cannot account for Stephanie's "devastation" at being unable to breastfeed her daughter for a full year (despite her recognition that Olive was unharmed), nor can they explain the class-privileged mothers in my study who pursued scientifically unsupported or potentially harmful "health" habits: highly restrictive fad diets, homeopathic remedies, and vaccine avoidance. Put another way, because the deficit model assumes that middle- and upper-class people's body-care practices will yield more desirable health outcomes, it cannot explain why those people might invest in medically unsound practices, nor can it explain why they might feel disappointment about achieving good health in the "wrong" way. And of course, the deficit model offers little insight into the potentially adaptive and beneficial practices that poor and working-class people engage in.

*The Reproduction of Inequality* explores a third explanation for class differences in health and body-care practices. I show how adopting so-called healthy lifestyles or consuming health products in the "right" way is a symbolic resource that can help mothers attain *cultural distinction*. *The Reproduction of Inequality* shows how, in their best efforts to care for their bodies and those of their children during pregnancy and postpartum, mothers display their own social status and transmit it to their children, reproducing social inequality through their very bodies.

## Maternal Bodies in Social Context

When we think about the stakes of body-care practices, we often focus on *individual* costs and benefits to health: Will a particular choice help us live longer, feel better, avoid costly medical interventions, or do more with our bodies? Indeed, these were the calculations women in my study described making, even as they arrived at different conclusions about which choices were worthwhile. *The Reproduction of Inequality* focuses instead on the *social* causes and consequences of maternal-health and body-care practices. Stories like Stephanie's and Gaby's might seem, at first glance, to operate on the microsocial level of personal habits, face-to-face social interactions, and all the various, everyday ways people learn to inhabit their bodies and present those bodies to others. Yet, the cumulative effect of these everyday practices adds up to something bigger than the individual, reflecting and reproducing inequality at the societal level. In this book, I use the case of maternal embodiment to understand two connected phenomena: (1) the stratification of bodies by ascribed social status, and (2) the cultural valuation of "health" as an achieved status, constituting both a personal and a public moral good.

### Stratified Embodiment

Bodies can become a resource for social status when some outward feature or ability gets commodified: a person with striking looks gets hired as a fashion model, or a person with unusual height, strength, or dexterity finds success as a professional athlete. Conversely, people whose bodies have significant functional impairments due to age, illness, or disability may struggle to find work if employers do not accommodate their bodies' limitations. But bodies factor into social inequality beyond their ability to labor or present a pleasing appearance. In the course of everyday social interaction, the body acts as a *visible symbol* of a person's ascribed status: the social group or position into which a person has been born or assigned.

Sometimes, these status groupings are treated as innate and essential, rooted in the body itself. Such is the case for systems of racial and gender inequality, where outward differences in the body's appearance get used as evidence for the "natural" superiority of one group over another.

Western medicine has long treated male bodies as the default or ideal form, and medical theories of the nineteenth century justified women's subordinate social position by claiming that (white) women were frail, sickly creatures at the mercy of their delicate reproductive organs.[4] Likewise, racist views within scientific and medical research have led scientists to conclude, at various points in history, that Black people have a greater tolerance for pain than whites, superior athletic ability, and—not coincidentally—a natural talent for manual labor.[5] These theories viewed white, male bodies as best suited to performing intellectual labor and holding positions of social power and responsibility while naturalizing the lower social status of women and people of color (as well as immigrants, people with disabilities, and other marginalized groups). Such racist and sexist ideologies refer back to the body in two ways. First, they justify social inequality as inevitable by treating the differences between sexes or races as essential and immutable, the result of inborn genetic differences in temperament, strength, intelligence, and so on. Second, these beliefs assign people to groups on the basis of observable differences like skin color or secondary sex characteristics: outward features that have little direct relation to the traits that supposedly differentiate races or sexes. These rather arbitrary outward signs become socially relevant because they are thought to signal a person's membership in a group believed to be biologically distinct.

In other systems of bodily stratification, physical appearance signifies not what kind of body one was born with but, rather, what one has *done* with it. Here, the body acts as a kind of visual record of the lives we have lived: the body bears witness in the form of scars, stretch marks, frown lines, and more. Habits like nail biting or regular dental care manifest on the body; musculature and posture can hint at how we spend our work and leisure time; and styling choices encompassing everything from haircuts to clothing, tattoos to cosmetic surgery, telegraph how we wish to present ourselves to others. Class, as an embodied system of social stratification, falls squarely within this second category of bodily signification: the class body expresses the uses to which one has put it, the cultural tastes in recreation and consumption that have shaped it, and the resources one has invested in it. Pierre Bourdieu, who coined the term "class bodies," explains, "The body is the most indisputable materialization of class taste, which it manifests in several ways. It does this first in the seemingly most natural features of the body, the dimensions (volume, height, weight) and shapes (round or square, stiff or supple, straight or curved) of its visible forms, which express in countless ways a whole relation to the body, i.e., a way of treating it, caring for it, feeding it, maintaining it, which reveals the deepest dispositions of the habitus."[6]

In sum, as biologist Anne Fausto-Sterling puts it, "Our bodies physically imbibe culture."[7] Class bodies are socially significant not just because of their direct consequences for a person's health and well-being but because of what they signify. They enable us to fit into certain social settings and not others, and they signal to observers where we belong: our habitus. And while our practices of "treating [the body], caring for it, feeding it, maintaining it" might seem, at first glance, to be a matter of individual effort or preferences, our class of origin plays an important role in shaping our attitudes toward our bodies and their use.

How do bodies become differentiated along class cultural lines in this way? Bourdieu argues that class differences in the use and care of bodies result from the interplay between material conditions and cultural tastes in consumption. People living with limited financial resources develop a "taste of necessity" wherein they come to appreciate and prefer those things (foods, leisure activities, entertainment) they can afford; members of wealthier classes develop a "taste of luxury."[8] While the taste of luxury often entails a preference for expensive or rare things, its defining feature is that it presumes freedom of choice: the ability to consume purely on the basis of taste, unconstrained by financial limitations. Thus, people with a taste of luxury might eschew costly but mass-market products in favor of items that cost relatively little but represent exclusivity in other ways (being local or handcrafted, requiring a discerning palate to enjoy, etc.).

For Bourdieu, the "taste of necessity" that shapes lower-income people's class bodies derives from their financial circumstances. Yet, because those circumstances are transformed into a cultural *taste*—which comes to be viewed as freely chosen and tied to one's values and priorities— the class body becomes the basis for moral judgments about members of a class. In this way, the highly cultivated body of the middle class "is spontaneously perceived as an index of moral uprightness, so that its opposite, a 'natural' body, is seen as an index of *laisser-aller* ('letting oneself go'), a culpable surrender to facility."[9] In short, poor and working-class people are more likely to be blamed for "letting themselves go"—for having bodies that are closer to nature and out of their personal control—while middle- and upper-class people are credited with having bodies that are carefully cultured, cultivated, and controlled. This binary that pits controlled, high-status bodies against "natural," out-of-control, and low-status bodies has long been used to justify a variety of social hierarchies, including man/woman, adult/child, white/nonwhite, colonizer/colonized, and more. These same symbolic meanings get mapped onto class bodies to naturalize class inequality. In essence, bodily differences across classes come to be understood not just as different but as *better* and *worse*.

### Health as a Stratified Moral Good

Race, gender, and class are all, for the most part, ascribed statuses: characteristics and group memberships assigned to us, rather than chosen or earned. In the United States, however, one of the most deeply held—if seldom fully realized—ideals is the notion that people should be judged according to their merits, not the circumstances of their birth. The aforementioned racist, sexist, and classist evaluations of some bodies as inherently better or worse than others do appear in US culture, but such beliefs conflict with meritocratic ideology. Yet, while meritocracy might frown on judging people for the bodies and circumstances they were born into, it does allow for judging people for what they do with—and to—those bodies. The bodily outcomes of people's work on—or neglect of—their appearance, health, and physical ability thus become an *achieved status*; here, the body signifies the individual's will power and personal character.

Or does it? As Bourdieu notes, cultural capital—the knowledge, tastes, and dispositions a society holds in high esteem—appears, at first glance, as merit. Cultural capital is typically formalized through educational credentials. Those credentials attest to the bearer as someone who has put in the time and effort to master difficult skills and knowledges, and they function as a key to unlocking high-status jobs and careers. Yet, while educational attainment requires work, it also advantages people whose family members are also highly educated, who can afford to hire tutors or attend private schools, and who can focus on school full-time instead of having to work or care for others. Thus, Bourdieu concludes, cultural-capital-as-education "manages to combine the prestige of innate property with the merits of acquisition. Because the social conditions of its transmission and acquisition are more disguised than those of economic capital, it is . . . unrecognized as capital and recognized as legitimate competence."[10] In this way, cultural capital, in the form of educational credentials, *launders* inherited financial privilege and makes it appear as individual merit. In the contemporary United States, "health" and health-related behaviors have come to function in much the same way.

Of course, the cultural valuation of health-promoting behaviors— and cultural scorn for those who squander their good health—is nothing new. Talcott Parsons, writing in 1951, described the "sick role" as a temporary status granted to those in ill health excusing them from their usual obligations in exchange for their earnest attempts to get better quickly.[11] To feign illness or to engage in behaviors that put oneself and others at risk would breach that social contract. What is fairly new, however, is the elevation of "health" to a primary societal value, "a metaphor for all that is good in life": an ideology known as "healthism."[12] Some scholars have likened healthism to a religion, wherein the pursuit of "health" is a moral obligation to which people must repeatedly demonstrate their devotion.[13] Healthism also aligns with neoliberal capitalist values, demanding that individuals invest in and optimize their bodies' functioning. In this era, writes Wendy Brown, "individuals [are seen] as rational, calculating creatures whose moral autonomy is measured by their capacity for 'self-care'—the ability to provide for their own needs and service their own ambitions."[14]

Robert Crawford traces the rise of healthism in the United States to the late 1970s, when middle-class people, in particular, began jogging, quitting smoking, and consuming all manner of health-related publications and other products.[15] During that time, "health" became more than just the absence of illness; it became a lifestyle and, for some, a source of cultural distinction. Indeed, I refer to "health" in quotation marks here because what we perceive as "healthy" is not always what is best for our well-being. Someone who loses weight due to cancer or an eating disorder may, nonetheless, receive compliments from coworkers for "getting healthy." Stephanie Brewer, quoted at the beginning of this chapter, agonized over failing to follow public health recommendations that she breastfeed her daughter for a year, even though her daughter was strong, happy, and developing typically. As Jonathan Metzl writes in the introduction to the provocatively named *Against Health*, "'Health' is a term replete with value judgments, hierarchies, and blind assumptions that speak as much about power and privilege as they do about well-being. Health is a desired state, but it is also a prescribed state and an ideological position."[16]

Under healthism, "health" and the attitudes and behaviors associated with its pursuit are *stratifying*: people who adopt "healthy" lifestyles and perform their devotion by talking about and consuming "health" projects in the right way are seen as morally superior to those who do not. In this way, "health" becomes an achieved status. But, as this book demonstrates, "health" is also *stratified*: people's participation in certain body-care practices and discourses is shaped by class and other preexisting inequalities. I show that, just as members of the privileged classes use education to transmit advantage to their children while disguising that advantage as merit, so too do they perform and transmit culturally esteemed body-care knowledges and practices in the earliest years of children's lives. In so doing, class-privileged people—mothers, specifically—ensure that their children will have the means to excel as morally worthy, "healthy" subjects.

## The Case of Maternal Embodiment

*The Reproduction of Inequality* examines these trends in the social valuation and stratification of bodies using the case of pregnant and postpartum women.[17] Pregnancy, childbirth, and breastfeeding represent an intensely embodied set of experiences. Major changes in the body itself—its size, center of gravity, felt sensations, and more—make most pregnant people hyperconscious of their bodies during this period. Additionally, social and medical norms demand that women monitor their bodies for signs of pregnancy, that they make significant changes in everyday health behaviors during and after pregnancy, and that they seek out medical oversight and education to learn yet more about their changing bodies. And surveillance by authorities and passersby—a coworker's comment on a pregnant woman's weight gain, for example, or a stranger's sidelong glance at someone breastfeeding in a public park— further contributes to body consciousness during this period.

On one hand, maternal embodiment—that period when the parent's body is directly sustaining the life of a fetus or newborn—might be said to represent a unique biological status, limited in duration and characterized by fairly unusual bodily circumstances. On the other hand, given social norms that valorize the pursuit of health and judge people according to the care they take of their bodies, maternal embodiment differs from "normal" embodiment in intensity more than in type. Women are socialized to work on their bodies through diet and exercise long before they have children: to maintain a conventionally attractive appearance, to demonstrate self-control and a dedicated work ethic, and to show their commitment to norms of "wellness" and risk awareness (even as the rewards for such work are mediated by color and class).[18] Pregnancy guidebooks, parenting apps for smartphones, and so-called mommy groups facilitate the transfer of these habits over to the maternal body once these women have children. Thus, many of the social values, norms, and processes that affect pregnant and breastfeeding bodies are the same as the ones that affect nonpregnant, nonbreastfeeding bodies. The *intensification* of those values, norms, and processes during maternal embodiment makes this period an ideal case study for understanding bodies in social context.

As later chapters show, social norms for the care of maternal and child bodies are bound up with gender roles, parenting ideologies, and more. Engaging with the large volume of sociological literature on motherhood has been fundamental to my understandings of maternal embodiment, and I see this project as contributing to that conversation. Yet, it is my hope that readers who have never been pregnant or given birth will be able to relate to my subjects' stories, too. We all have bodies; we all live in social settings where our bodies are subject to norms for how we should look or behave; and we all, to varying degrees, must learn to care for and make sense of our bodies in light of those norms.

## Methods and Participants

To understand mothers' body-care practices in social context, I focused on two levels of analysis: first, the institutional and historical norms that define what "good" maternal and child body care looks like during and after pregnancy; second, the individual-level meanings that mothers attached to their bodily practices and experiences. In this way, I aimed to capture both the top-down and bottom-up processes through which maternal body care reflects and reproduces inequality.

## Sites

I conducted in-depth interviewing and ethnography in two geographic regions of the United States: the San Francisco Bay Area in Northern California, and the inland, north-central region of Florida. The Bay Area, where I launched this project, is known for being on the forefront of national food and health trends. Numerous local writers and restaurateurs (including Alice Waters, Michael Pollan, and Thomas Keller) have become trendsetters in the areas of "slow," local, and organic eating, and innovative state-level public health policies like indoor smoking bans, helmet laws, and emissions regulations have become models for other states to emulate. Given these local factors, I suspected that research subjects in the Bay Area might be more health and body conscious than women in other parts of the country. For this reason, I decided to add a second research site, ultimately settling on a region in north-central Florida near the Georgia border. This location was characterized by laxer public health laws (such as the requirement that motorcycle riders wear a helmet *only* if they were under twenty-one or lacked insurance), and the local cuisine was dominated by casual drinking and dining establishments (during my time there, the local newspaper ran multiple features excitedly announcing the opening of a Five Guys burger restaurant).

As a qualitative study, this project was not designed to be statistically generalizable to the United States as a whole; nonetheless, in studying these two regions comparatively, I hoped to get a better sense of major trends in maternal embodiment overall, as well as to see how they played out in divergent local contexts. In each state, I was based in a city with a large, public university and frequently drove up to an hour in order to reach mothers living in outlying rural and suburban areas. Additionally, both states boasted impressive agricultural economies: California is the single largest agricultural producer in the United States, and Florida is one of the top producers of fruit and vegetable crops. Furthermore, due to their agricultural production and temperate climates, California and Florida ranked among the top states to have winter farmers' markets in 2010 (placing second and fourth out of all fifty states, respectively). These factors may have given women in my study greater-than-average year-round access to fresh fruits and vegetables, enabling them to have more nutritious eating habits than people in some other parts of the country.[19]

Apart from these similarities, though, I selected these two regions on the basis of several key differences. In California, I based my research in a politically progressive metropolitan area (known for its liberal politics even within a historically Democratic-voting state), while my Florida research site was located within a politically conservative region of a "purple" state that trended Republican. Demographics were also important, with the California site being multiethnic and urban, while the Florida site was—with the exception of the university town itself— highly rural and characterized by a largely Black-white racial makeup. The southeast region of the United States tends to have the country's lowest rates of breastfeeding and maternity care, while the West is strongest on these measures.[20] Furthermore, in contrast with the highbrow "foodie" culture of the Bay Area, my Florida site was, both culturally and geographically speaking, a part of the southeastern United States. Poor whites in the region proudly referred to themselves as "crackers" (a sometimes-pejorative term that, when used in this way, connotes that one is a local). And subjects from middle- and lower-class backgrounds alike referenced family traditions of southern comfort foods like boiled peanuts, fried chicken, and grits.

## Recruitment and Participant Observation

Throughout 2010 and 2011, I conducted one-time, in-depth interviews with women in Florida and California. I used a prewritten interview schedule of open-ended questions to guide the conversation, with questions ordered more or less chronologically: beginning with questions about what was going on in subjects' lives when they first learned they were pregnant and moving through their experiences of being pregnant, giving birth, and infant feeding, and ending with questions about their hopes for the body-care values and habits their children would learn as they grew older. Follow-up questions asked women to elaborate on their beliefs and preferences, as well as to discuss their relationship to various sources of support and information (such as peers, family members, medical providers, and parenting books). Not all women were asked all of the questions—for example, those who were currently pregnant with their first child were unable to answer questions about infant feeding—and conversations sometimes departed from the order of the interview schedule in order to follow up on themes that subjects introduced.

I recruited participants through a variety of local organizations catering to the needs of new and expectant mothers. To make contact with middle- and upper-class mothers, I received moderators' permission to post flyers for my project on regional Internet communities for parents, all of which had highly active memberships, organized local events for mothers, and provided forums, message boards, and web links for parenting support. I also took advantage of invitations to come observe in-person meetings of two activity and support groups for mothers: in Florida, an area meeting of La Leche League (a support group for breastfeeding mothers and their children) and, in California, a "baby boot camp" exercise program for new mothers trying to establish regular exercise routines after giving birth. In each, I gave a short presentation on my project and handed out my contact information to women who expressed interest in participating; I also carried out informal participant observation, exercising or completing worksheet-based activities alongside the mothers and—when feasible—having casual conversations with mothers about their participation in this and other mothers' groups. I conducted my interviews with these women outside of the group setting and—when we had finished—I initiated snowball sampling, asking them to pass my name on to other women they knew who might wish to participate. I recruited roughly equal numbers of women through my initial contacts in listservs and mothers' groups and through follow-up snowball sampling, for a total of thirty-six. In one case, an interview I had planned as a one-on-one discussion became an impromptu joint interview with two mothers when my interviewee—Cass Blackwell—invited a friend from her postpartum support group to join us.

Neither the in-person support groups for mothers nor the online communities were formally limited to middle- and upper-class mothers, although the "baby boot camp" did require an enrollment fee. However, it was difficult to reach poor and working-class women through these sites; of the thirty-six women I recruited in this way, thirty ultimately ended up in the high-education, high-income category of my study. In order to target low-income mothers, I conducted recruitment and participant observation in offices of the Women, Infants, and Children (WIC) program. WIC is a federal, means-tested program run by the US Food and Nutrition Service but administered largely at the state and local levels. WIC provides food and nutrition assistance to low-income women, infants, and children who are at or below 185 percent of the federal poverty line.[21] WIC recipients participate in group or one-on-one nutrition counseling as a condition of their enrollment, and they receive voucher coupons that they can exchange for foods like milk, cheese, bread, and produce at participating grocery stores. I selected eight total offices from which to recruit women for interviews: four offices in different counties in the San Francisco Bay Area, and four offices in different counties in rural northern Florida. I spent about a week of nonconsecutive days at each of the eight sites, observing nutrition-education classes and one-on-one counseling sessions, building rapport with clients (often by offering to play with their children while they completed WIC paperwork), and conducting interviews with staff members during down time.[22] I also handed out short surveys to mothers sitting in the waiting rooms and gave them the option of listing their name and phone number if they would be willing to be interviewed. Seventy-five percent of the women agreed to be contacted. I called them at home and, of those, I ended up conducting in-depth interviews with thirty-four women in their homes, in cafés, and in public parks and playgrounds.

## A Note about "Mothers"

Throughout this book, I will refer to my subjects as "women" or "mothers." All of the people I interviewed identified as women, all had conceived and carried their own biological offspring, and all were raising or intending to raise those children. In other words, they were biologically, socially, and personally identified as mothers. For the purposes of my research, I sought subjects who had firsthand experiences with the physiological processes of conceiving and bearing children and who faced the gendered social norms that govern women raising children.

That said, not everyone who mothers is the biological parent of a child, and not everyone who gives birth to a child identifies as a mother. I use the term "mother" for the sake of brevity and to mirror the language my subjects used to describe themselves, but readers should not assume that my findings necessarily apply to all people who mother or who have given birth.

## Participants

The women I interviewed represented a wide range of ages, life experiences, racial/ethnic backgrounds, and class positions (see the appendix for a full list). I developed my initial class categorizations on the basis of whether or not subjects were eligible for WIC. This classification scheme shaped my recruitment efforts: because WIC serves roughly half of all American households with young children, this cutoff served as a handy divider between the upper and lower socioeconomic halves of my sample. I classified WIC-eligible mothers as "low income," which corresponded, approximately, to falling into the first or second quintile of all US households in 2011 (annual household incomes of $0–38,520). Most WIC-ineligible mothers I spoke to—my "high-income" sample— fell into the fourth or fifth quintiles for household income ($62,435 or higher per year).[23] However, the questions I wanted to ask about class and the body dealt with more than socioeconomic status. I wanted to know about class cultural differences, too, and so I further categorized mothers on the basis of educational attainment: "high education" women were those who had completed a four-year college degree or higher; "low education" women had not. Here, educational attainment serves as a proxy for class differences in cultural capital.[24]

Past research demonstrates the tight links between education and the possession of highly valued tastes, habits, and knowledges (cultural capital). Children who inherit high-status cultural capital from their families typically find an easier "fit" with behavioral and social norms in school, enabling them to build better relationships with teachers and understand what is expected of them.[25] These children go on to have higher levels of educational attainment generally and college attendance specifically.[26] Earning a college degree is thus strongly correlated with the possession of inherited cultural capital. More recently, Anthony Jack found that while cultural capital matters for college success, it need not only be inherited from one's family: poor students who attended even one year of elite college preparatory school showed similar levels of ease in navigating college cultural norms and pursuing opportunities as their wealthier peers.[27] Whether cultural capital is acquired in early childhood or later on, it remains a strong predictor of college completion; possession of a college degree thus signals one's fluency with middle-class cultural and professional norms.

For the majority of women, educational status and economic status were closely connected: thirty respondents were high-education, high-income (henceforth "HH") and twenty-six were low-education, low-income ("LL"). However, fourteen respondents did not fit neatly into this class dichotomy. These "mixed-class" mothers, as I call them, included eight highly educated women with low household incomes (HL) and six lower-education women with relatively high household incomes (LH). Many of these mixed-class women had experienced upward or downward mobility relative to their classes of origin. Some were on an upward trajectory: becoming the first in their family to attend college or building a successful business. Others had experienced downward mobility, though that status might be temporary: a college-educated couple whose household incomes had plummeted after one partner decided to attend graduate school or to become a stay-at-home parent.

Although this heterogeneous "mixed-class" group was not part of my original research plan, over time I came to realize their importance to the project. They, perhaps more than any other group, illuminate how class matters as a cause and consequence of women's maternal body projects. Throughout the book, there are two features of this group that I will return to. First, mixed-class people possess conflicting class markers, being either high education/low income (HL) or low education/high income (LH). Comparing their attitudes, rhetoric, and practices to the high/high and low/low groups helps us understand which dimension of class is responsible for a particular class-differentiated pattern: if financial resources drive some behavior, then we would expect high-income women (whether college educated or not) to behave one way and low-income women to behave another. If, however, class cultural norms and knowledges are the cause, then mixed-class women with college or graduate degrees will likely resemble their higher-income, college-educated peers. In short, mixed-class women can help us understand the extent to which class differences in health and body care are due to cultural or material forces.

Second, mixed-class mothers are more likely than most other women to have mixed social contacts: family members and acquaintances who are significantly higher or lower income (or education) than themselves. These contacts made them more aware of class differences in knowledge and practices than most other mothers—and also, perhaps, more anxious to draw sharp distinctions between themselves and lower-status peers. HH and LL mothers took part in class-differentiated health and body-care practices, but they rarely spoke explicitly about their choices in terms of class. Mixed-class mothers, however, were among the most likely to understand the class implications of their choices, and the most likely to talk about them.

Women from these three class groupings—HH, LL, and mixed-class—looked markedly different from one another. High-education, high-income mothers ranged in age from their late twenties to early forties, with an average age of thirty-one when they had their first child. Many HH women worked in professional careers, though several had reduced their work hours or had become stay-at-home parents once their children were born. All were married to the fathers of their children and lived in single-family homes with just their husbands and children (none self-identified as lesbian or bisexual). Though most were financially comfortable, this varied by age and location: younger couples, including a few in which one or both partners were enrolled in graduate school, tended to have high future earnings prospects but were currently living on modest budgets; older couples had at least one spouse with a high-earning professional career, owned their own homes, and had a high amount of disposable income. Not all HH mothers had intended to become pregnant when they did, but most of these women's pregnancies were planned; several also shared stories about medically assisted reproductive procedures like in vitro fertilization that they had used to become pregnant. Nearly all (twenty-six out of thirty) of my HH respondents identified as white; the four nonwhite respondents self-identified as Asian, Latina, or biracial (white/Asian or white/Latina).

In contrast, most low-education, low-income mothers were unmarried and relatively young: averaging about twenty-one when they had their first child, a decade younger than their HH counterparts. Women in this group typically had a high school diploma or GED, and some were pursuing associate's or bachelor's degrees when I spoke to them. Though usually unmarried, some LL women had male partners with whom they cohabited. Others lived in households with members of their extended families: their own parents, perhaps one or more of their siblings, and their siblings' children. These extended family households combined resources and mutual support in a variety of ways, pooling paychecks, childcare duties, and benefits from public assistance programs like WIC, welfare, SNAP (food stamps), and more. Poor and working-class women were more likely to experience their pregnancies as an interruption of their plans (for education or financial independence) than as the result of careful planning. Women in this group were racially and ethnically diverse: almost half (twelve out of twenty-six) were Black, ten were white, and four were Latina.

Mixed-class women, not surprisingly, fell in between these two class groups: they averaged age twenty-eight when they had their first child, and hailed from every income quintile except for the first (lowest-income) quintile. Three of the white mothers in this group were unmarried; the three nonwhite mothers (two Asian, one Latina) were all married. Because of this group's heterogeneity, the lifestyles of mixed-class mothers are hard to generalize, but later chapters will tease out some of the ways these women navigated between class positions.

Lastly, while class was one main focus of my sampling, I also looked for patterns according to region and race/ethnicity. With regard to region, I recruited similar numbers of respondents from the two states in my study: forty-one mothers from Florida, twenty-nine from California, with similar proportions falling into each of the three class groupings. Yet, despite the demographic and political differences in these two geographic regions, I was struck by the similarities I heard in women's stories; for this reason, in subsequent chapters I will not routinely highlight geographic patterns in my findings. More challenging was the task of exploring racial/ethnic patterns in women's responses. While I tried various strategies to recruit an ethnically diverse sample, it remained the case that most of my HH respondents were white, and more than half of my LL respondents were not. To the extent that such comparisons are possible with this sample, I have looked carefully for racial/ethnic differences in response patterns. Where my own empirical data are lacking—most notably, the absence of Black women in my mixed-class and HH groups—I draw on the work of other scholars to provide a fuller picture of how interactions between race and class (what Maxine Leeds Craig calls "racialized class") play out on the body.[28]

### Rapport and Researcher Subjectivity

I conducted interviews for this project as a childless woman in my late twenties. I was married, but took off my wedding ring for interviews because I did not want to invite questions about my own family status. Specifically, I did not want to field questions about my "husband" and be forced either to lie or to come out as queer (I did not assume my respondents would be homophobic, but I also wanted to minimize the chance that my identity would be a distraction). Nevertheless, many respondents wanted to know if I had had children, and my usual response was a cheerful, "Not yet!" In responding this way, I hoped to communicate to interviewees that they had expert, firsthand knowledge and I was there to learn from them. I had no preconceived notions about the "best" way to feed and care for a baby since I had not yet had to make those decisions myself (thus, I was less likely to judge them). In short, I invited them to view me as a potential future mother who could benefit from their hard-won wisdom.

This was a strategic positioning I adopted to build rapport, but I had no idea at the time how accurate my framing of the relationship would become. While writing this book, I became pregnant with my first child. Reviewing interview transcripts, I would sometimes pause to look down at my belly, rippling with movement. Reading mothers' accounts of pregnancy risks or parenting resources often sent me down a rabbit hole of Internet searching (not unlike many of the highly educated, self-described "control freak" moms I interviewed); as I read and took classes in preparation for childbirth, I became better attuned to picking up on key terms my interviewees were using, as when one respondent described reframing labor as "intense" rather than "painful," which I could now identify as a catch phrase of "natural childbirth" proponents like midwife/author Ina May Gaskin. Most of all, however, I felt lucky beyond measure to be heading into parenthood with the combined wisdom of seventy mothers to guide me. Unlike many mothers-to-be, I have gotten to hear—in great, intimate detail—from both women demographically similar to me (white, highly educated, older first-time parents) and those whose experiences and backgrounds are very different from my own, all of which have afforded me a valuable sense of proportion.

If there is one personal lesson that I have been able to take from all of these women's stories, it is this: babies survive and thrive under a wide variety of conditions. Some are born in hospitals, others at home; some women exclusively breastfeed, others supplement or feed entirely with formula; some babies are cared for solely by their parents while others spend many hours of their day in paid childcare or with extended family and friends. Although it is the argument of this book that class-differentiated body-care practices *accumulate* to produce distinct class bodies (with consequences for mothers' and children's social status), it also became apparent to me that the consequences of any *one* parenting decision are usually minimal. I wish I could say that this realization cured me of all desire to micromanage my own body during and after pregnancy. As my spouse, Jen, can attest, it did not. But I do think that it lent me a sense of humor about the process, an ability to step back, take a deep breath, and remember that healthy, happy babies come into the world in many different ways. For this, I am forever indebted to the women who shared their time and stories with me.

## Organization of the Book

In the chapters that follow, I elaborate different pieces of my central argument: namely, that in the contemporary United States, the care and cultivation of the body have become critical means through which social status is maintained and transmitted, and that this process is particularly intensified for new mothers and their children.

Chapter 1 introduces the concept of *reproductive body projects*: the set of everyday body-care practices women undertook to cultivate babies' development by working on their own maternal bodies during and after pregnancy. While bodies are physical and biological, they are also social; we learn to care for, use, and make meaning out of our bodies in community with others. The composition of that community varies, however, by class. HH mothers, I found, sought advice and support through *horizontal* relationships with peers and healthcare providers who shared their values, where they could demonstrate their expertise. LL women were more likely to rely on *vertical* relationships with health authorities and their own mothers, putting their faith in people with more experience or specialized knowledge than themselves.

In chapters 2 and 3, I look at the social norms and expectations guiding women's assumption of responsibility for health and body care within their families. Chapter 2 examines the gendered patterns of responsibility that cut across class lines. Nurturing children's developing bodies requires a series of related competencies: *noticing* a child's needs, tastes, and desires; *gathering information* about health and developmental issues as they arise; and *supervising* husbands, babysitters, and other helpers in providing care. Women's ability to perform these tasks was not innate but rather, it was the result of years of practice. Most mothers traced their knowledge of dieting, nutrition, risk avoidance, and more to their pre-pregnancy body-care regimens. Already well versed in the gendered practice of "doing health" (which links bodily self-care to femininity), these women learned to extend their body consciousness to their children and families.

Chapter 3 presents the two frameworks that women in my study used to make decisions about health and body care. The hegemonic *risk-avoidant paradigm* seeks to promote child well-being at all costs and minimize all risks, however slight; the alternative *risk-assessing paradigm*, in contrast, is one in which women act as informed consumers of health information, calculating risks to their children while balancing them against other personal and household priorities. Yet while all women found themselves judged against the risk-avoidant paradigm— and all occasionally had to find compromises between what was ideal and what was possible—the consequences of failing to live up to the risk-avoidant ideal were not borne equally. HH white women, in particular, often received the benefit of the doubt, sometimes even receiving permission to relax their vigilance (as in the case of doctors who "prescribed" them a glass of wine). LL women, on the other hand, faced constant scrutiny and second guessing; for these mothers, the "no cost is too great" approach to parenting was both financially prohibitive and socially compulsory to avoid being viewed as "bad mothers."

Chapters 4 and 5 use narrative analysis, a method for interpreting subjects' stories as intentionally constructed *narratives* that subjects use to understand and communicate something about themselves to an audience. Chapter 4 examines how women across classes did—or did not—connect their body-care choices during and after pregnancy to a larger sense of self-identity. HH women, I found, drew strong and frequent connections between their reproductive body projects and their self-identities. They identified as particular types of eaters, as athletes, or as accomplished professionals, and they often went to great lengths to reconcile inconsistencies in their histories in order to present a coherent picture of their identities as individuals committed to managing their own health and wellness. LL women, in contrast, frequently resisted making their self-care practices the basis for an identity. The *disidentification* they engaged in—accepting the value of mainstream health norms even as they framed those norms as burdensome or distasteful— illuminates the extent to which constructing a coherent self-identity requires the financial resources to consume personalized health products and services as well as class cultural fluency in the language of healthism.

Chapter 5 examines how changes in mothers' bodies—including episodes where their maternal bodies felt out of control—affected mothers' sense of agency. Women across classes experienced similar physical changes and challenges during pregnancy, childbirth, and the postpartum period, but they responded in different ways. For HH women, these changes represented a body that was potentially out of control, and most sought to reassert control over their bodies through what I call "*rigid agency*." In contrast, LL women responded to the twists and turns of new and expectant motherhood with *flexible agency*: they still made choices about their bodies and those of their children, but they focused less on rigidly determining an outcome and more on flexibly negotiating different alternatives. While both approaches represent class-conditioned responses to situational conditions, I argue that one—rigid agency—falls more in line with classical conceptions of agency and full personhood, but the other—flexible agency—is better suited to helping women adapt and thrive through the bodily changes of pregnancy and postpartum embodiment.

In chapter 6, I turn toward the future, asking how mothers' investments in their children's health and body-care habits today might reproduce class inequalities later in life—a form of care work I term "*status work*." Few women of any class explicitly framed their practices as designed to transmit class advantages. At most, they referred vaguely to practices aimed at giving children the "best start in life," and most spoke about the importance of teaching children to love and take care of their bodies. What that looked like, however, differed substantially across classes. HH mothers emphasized the social meanings of eating rituals; the importance of informed consumption; and the pursuit of moderation as a virtue. LL mothers, in contrast, highlighted cleanliness; the transmission of simple, easy-to-follow health rules; and the urgency of avoiding chronic illness and disability. On one hand, these differences certainly show class to be a *cause* of divergent health habits, a function of disparate resources and cultural contexts. On the other hand, I argue that class-specific modes of caring for the body can function as a form of embodied cultural capital, priming children to move into their parents' class and contributing to the process of social reproduction.

## Conclusion

Despite its focus on "health" and inequality, *The Reproduction of Inequality* is not, primarily, interested in comparing rates of actual death and disease between women of different class backgrounds. To be sure, these differences exist: wealthier people tend to live longer and to spend more of their years disease free relative to poorer people; racial/ethnic minority groups, especially Black and Indigenous people in the United States, are at higher risk of serious illness or death from causes ranging from diabetes to asthma, heart disease to COVID-19, preeclampsia to maternal mortality, even after controlling for socioeconomic status.[29] But, as voluminous research makes clear, these disparities cannot be explained by individual behaviors alone. Rather, they are the result of factors known, collectively, as the "social determinants of health": structural conditions such as exposure to air and water pollution; neighborhood safety or violence; accessible transportation and healthcare; affordable nutritious foods; occupational safety; and more.[30] The social determinants of health shape population well-being generally, and they matter particularly for maternal and infant health.

Yet, despite decades of evidence that disparities in maternal and infant health require structural solutions, advice to new mothers largely focuses on individual behaviors. Expectant mothers learn about the numerous harms that might result from consuming the wrong foods, exercising too much (or too little), sleeping in the wrong position, taking too much (or too little) medicine, and more. My interviews with women reveal that higher- and lower-status women respond differently to such advice, incorporating disparate practices into their reproductive body projects and attributing different meanings to those efforts. What, if not actual health and well-being, might be the effects of these differences?

I argue that mothers' reproductive body projects carry social as well as physiological consequences. The social burdens and benefits that mothers face when it comes to their care of their bodies illustrate the stratified workings of "health" and healthism in US society more broadly. Without exception, all of the women in my study took on reproductive body projects for the sake of their children's health and development. They did so out of a sense of loving obligation, but also because societal discourses about health dictated the lengths to which they must go to discharge that obligation. Explicitly, the goal of these projects is to optimize the biological processes of *human reproduction*, resulting in healthy children. Implicitly, as this book shows, these projects facilitate the long-term process of *social reproduction*, which makes it likely that children will inherit not only their parents' genes but their social class and culture as well.

1

# Maternal Embodiment

## *How Reproductive Body Projects Work*

Pregnancy, childbirth, and breastfeeding—the features of maternal embodiment that are this book's core focus—are bodily processes made possible by the workings of hormones, reproductive organs, and other physiological mechanisms. At the same time, these bodily processes are profoundly *social*: facilitated by a range of human-made medical technologies and techniques, taking place with unequal access to health resources and safe environments, and managed through social relationships that convey culture-specific ideas about the body and its care. The biology of human reproduction is fairly straightforward, shared across all members of the species who successfully conceive and bear children; the sociology of human reproduction, however, is considerably more variable. As women in my study interacted with friends, family members, and health professionals—and as they consumed a variety of media about maternal embodiment—they found that their bodies and practices were being observed, commented on, and measured against social norms for "good" embodiment. Such conversations were sometimes informative and empowering, at other times judgmental and unwelcome, and—to some extent—managed through women's decisions about which relationships to cultivate.

India Brown was a Black, twenty-year-old single mother (LL) living in California when I spoke with her in the home she shared with her mother, younger siblings, and one-year-old daughter.[1] She recounted the unsolicited advice she had received at her baby shower from a number of older family members and family friends: "They were like, 'You have to eat more,' because my legs were skinny. I had this big old huge belly, and they were like, 'Your legs are too skinny! You're not eating enough!' They were telling me all this stuff that I needed to eat, and I was just like, 'That's hecka rude.' And some other things that they would

tell me were 'Don't wear your shirts too tight.' . . . It was kind of annoy-
ing. . . . Old people—you know how they have old ideas about things!"
India discounted some of her friends' and relatives' comments on her
body as "hecka rude," outdated ideas coming from "old people." Yet
when it came to her daughter's health, she also sought out advice from
the people she trusted: "The first person I would go to is my mom. The
second person I would go to is probably my grandma. And the third
person is [my daughter's] doctor, because if after them two, after all the
kids they have raised, they don't know, then I probably need to go to a
doctor to talk about it."

India's mixed experiences with receiving advice about her own body
and her daughter's body are, in many ways, typical for women across
classes. Many women recounted to me the ways that their bodies became hypervisible during pregnancy, eliciting comments from friends
and strangers alike that often felt intrusive and rude. Accustomed to
thinking of their bodies as personal and private, most mothers viewed
the increasingly public status of their bodies as an unwelcome development. At the same time, the new physical experiences and sensations of
maternal embodiment—combined with women's near-universal desire
to make healthful choices for their baby's growth—led most women to
seek out advice and support through informal social networks and/or
via formal institutions they belonged to.

Lori Kent (HH), a white, twenty-nine-year-old mother of one living
in Florida, reflected on the challenges of navigating multiple, conflicting social norms that she had encountered while pregnant: "Different
people were amazed that I was still drinking caffeine [when I was preg-
nant]. Even though I was completely comfortable with it, there were
a couple of times where people who knew absolutely nothing about it
were like, 'Oh my gosh, you're still drinking coffee?' I'm like, it's one cup
a day. And they would be like, 'You've got to do everything possible for
your kid.'" Lori, a graduate student in biology, was irritated by what she
viewed as the outdated social norm that pregnant women should sacrifice all of their comforts, including caffeine. She explained, "I looked at
multiple studies that showed one cup a day did not make any difference.
It was frustrating. . . . I am kind of snobby about this, because I do this
research. I don't make a decision lightly. And then I feel like these people
who don't know as much as me make comments."

Like India, Lori did not make her body-care decisions in isolation; rather, she became used to dealing with unhelpful judgments and advice while simultaneously seeking out guidance from trusted sources. In claiming "I do this research," Lori did not mean that her graduate study focused on measuring the effects of caffeine. Like many women I spoke to, she used the term "research" to describe an informal process of gathering information from various sources: sometimes academic studies but also popular books and magazines, blog posts, medical providers, and more.

Lori also noted, with wry amusement, that she was equally as exasperated with unsolicited praise as she was with unwelcome judgments. When, in the weeks before she gave birth, acquaintances learned that she intended to breastfeed, she recalled how their responses surprised her: "[People would say] 'I'm so proud of you that you're planning on breastfeeding,' and it was kind of like, 'I'm not doing this to get your approval.'" Lori shook her head and chuckled, adding, "I never really engaged someone in a real conversation about it, except like my husband or my mom. . . . But it was still weird, because I got approval for things that I wasn't looking for approval for." Lori's discomfort with this approval came not because she lacked conviction in her choice to breastfeed but because these interactions revealed that her private choices were subject to very public scrutiny.

Lori's and India's stories illustrate how families, peer groups, medical professionals, and other individuals and institutions served a dual role in this process. On one hand, they provided mothers with support and information, helping women adjust to the unfamiliar bodily sensations of motherhood, and offering a reassuring answer to the worried question of many a new parent: "Is this normal?" On the other hand, these social networks and institutions often became sites of what Michel Foucault has called "normalizing judgment," measuring mothers' bodies and practices against an unspoken—and, sometimes, spoken—norm.[2] Such judgment demands that women engage in socially normative reproductive body projects, with others offering praise—or condemnation—on the basis of women's efforts. Women across classes are subject to this judgment, but while low-income women often must submit to judgmental surveillance in exchange for aid (including financial support both from family members and from the state), middle- and upper-class mothers more often claim for themselves the status of expert, resisting judgment and prioritizing social relationships where their health beliefs and practices will be validated.[3]

In this chapter, I look at the everyday social contexts within which mothers learned to care for their maternal bodies and the bodies of their children and to navigate the social scrutiny that accompanied this work. During and after pregnancy, women engage in what I call "reproductive body projects": a set of deliberately chosen and enacted body-care practices aimed at cultivating babies' development by working on the maternal body. The contents and contexts of these projects varied, but virtually all mothers were expected to engage in this work. In the sections that follow, I will examine how reproductive body projects are conceived of and situated in relation to social norms for the care and management of bodies. I then compare higher- and lower-class women's development of reproductive projects across three significant social relationships: with health experts; with their own mothers (children's grandmothers); and with peers.

## Normalizing Support and Judgment

Neither Lori nor India recalled explicitly being called "bad" mothers, but both felt that was the subtext of acquaintances' critical comments about their bodies. Indeed, pregnant and breastfeeding bodies are subject to a wide range of formal and informal surveillance in the contemporary United States: these bodies are judged for what they do or do not ingest, how readily they comply with medical directives, how much or little weight they gain, how they give birth, whether (and for how long) they breastfeed, and more. In many ways, maternal embodiment draws an intensified version of the scrutiny all bodies face in this health-focused society, with women expected to manage their bodies through carefully cultivated *reproductive body projects*. And because the standards for "good" maternal body care are multiple, contradictory, and often unattainable, no one is fully safe from judgment.

On one hand, then, mothers in all classes face social pressure to make good choices for their own health and their children's health and to avoid risk, which—as I will discuss in the next chapter—represents a particularly *gendered* social imperative. On the other hand, the social resources through which women learn about body-care norms and seek support for their choices differ significantly by class (and, to some extent, by race/ethnicity as well). As this chapter will show, poor and working-class women drew support mainly from close, personal relationships with their mothers and trusted health authorities like pediatricians and WIC counselors. Middle- and upper-class women, in contrast, tended to favor peers and independent inquiry. Put another way, lower-status (LL) women tended to access support and information through *vertical* relationships in which they looked to someone with more experience or expertise for guidance; higher-status (HH) women instead sought out and established *horizontal* relationships, seeking to become knowledge experts in their own right and interacting with doctors and other health professionals more or less as equals. Through these moves, class-privileged women asserted their moral status as health entrepreneurs and their social status as equal—not subordinate—to health experts. Poor and working-class women, on the other hand, often judged themselves—and were judged by others—as having insufficient knowledge or commitment to health, which positioned them as passive recipients of information from health professionals and more experienced mothers. In this way, middle- and upper-class mothers' reproductive body projects—more than those of poor and working-class women—become resources for asserting a high, achieved social status.

## Reproductive Body Projects

Women like India and Lori were held accountable to performing a particular kind of work on their bodies and health attitudes in the process of becoming mothers. Sociologists use the term "body projects" to describe this work more generally. Writes Chris Shilling, "In the West in particular, there is a tendency for the body to be seen as an entity in the process of becoming; a project to be worked at and accomplished as part of an individual's self-identity. . . . Treating the body as a project . . . involve[s] individuals being conscious of, and actively concerned about, the management and appearance of their bodies."[4] Body projects, which commonly include practices like dieting, fitness regimens, sport- or occupation-specific physical training, consumption of medical technologies, and more, assert not only that our bodies *can* be altered through our deliberate actions but also that they *should*. The reasons for this imperative vary, but often include a sense of obligation to one's family or community (to remain healthy and productive), as well as a moral charge to avoid the appearance of laziness, complacency, or letting oneself go. Fundamentally, body projects position the body's ability and appearance as elements of an achieved status.

The work that women in my study described doing, which I term "reproductive body projects," often represented an extension of their pre-pregnancy body projects, but these projects also involved a number of specialized practices tied to the liminal bodily states of pregnancy and breastfeeding, wherein the boundaries between maternal and child bodies are porous. Reproductive body projects, then, can be defined as a set of deliberately chosen and enacted body-care practices that aim to provide an optimal environment for fetal development during pregnancy; to support safe and successful childbirth; and, postpartum, to provide balanced infant nutrition (often through breastfeeding) while simultaneously returning the mother's body to a healthy nonpregnant state. The specific contents of reproductive body projects are shaped by scientific information about health as well as by ideology. As the following sections show, class and other cultural groupings significantly shaped women's notions of which health and body-care practices were *optimal*, while material opportunities and constraints further influenced which practices were *possible*. What linked women across classes was the expectation that they should take on these projects, that they looked to others to help them learn about and navigate the work that these projects required, and that they faced evaluation on the basis of those projects.

## Connecting with Health Professionals and Expert Advice

The majority of women considered medical advice carefully when they were making decisions about how to care for their bodies during pregnancy or postpartum. Once relatively common experiences overseen by lay practitioners and family members, pregnancy and childbirth in the United States today have been *medicalized*: viewed through the lens of health and subjected to oversight by medical experts.[5] Social and medical norms call for the regular monitoring of fetal development even in seemingly uneventful pregnancies, and pregnant and breastfeeding people are regularly urged to "consult your doctor" before taking medication or engaging in physically demanding activities. For the most part, women in my study did consult medical sources: physicians and licensed midwives, WIC and other public health workers, and scientific publications. Mothers did not always dutifully follow this advice, but overall, medical norms for the correct care of the maternal (and child) body dominated these women's decisions.

### "You build up a relationship with these people": Poor and Working-Class Mothers and Health Authorities

Vanessa Garfield (white, twenty-five, LL) was a married mother of two living in Florida when I met her. Vanessa's husband had a job at Walmart, and Vanessa was working toward an associate's degree at a nearby community college while acting as primary caregiver to their young sons, aged two and four. For her family, WIC aid mattered both because it supplemented their household budget with vouchers for free food and, as Vanessa recounted, because her counselor taught her to do more with the food they had. As Vanessa explained, "[WIC has] been really good, especially with my older son, because we had a really hard time getting him to eat vegetables. So [the nutritionist] gave us a lot of different ways that we could introduce it to him, and a lot of different choices that we could offer, and it seemed to help. So now he is eating his vegetables." When I asked how the nutritionist talked to her about this issue, Vanessa responded, "She gave us a grid of different ones that he should have every day. She talked to him about it and got him to want to try stuff." Vanessa saw her WIC counselor as a trustworthy and effective source of information, particularly when it came to addressing her son's pickiness.

Another mother, Lynne O'Brien (white, twenty-seven, LL), also had positive experiences with WIC. Her youngest, a three-year-old daughter, was eligible for WIC, but the whole household—including Lynne and her husband, their two older sons (ages six and eight), and Lynne's mother and brother—benefited from the infusion of free, nutritious foods. WIC policy does not prohibit household members from sharing in these benefits, but it differs from some other food-assistance programs like SNAP (formerly known as "food stamps") in that it is highly prescriptive about which foods the benefit covers. Diya, a nutritionist at one Florida WIC office I visited, explained the updated food voucher system that WIC debuted in 2009: "Food packages provide milk, cheese, eggs, juice, cereal. We offer a whole grain food voucher—whole wheat bread, brown rice, or corn tortillas—and then a fruit and vegetable voucher up to a certain dollar amount. For prenatal [clients], it is ten dollars a month, then for children, it's six dollars. And they can buy fresh, frozen, or canned fruits and vegetables as long as they're not seasoned."

WIC clients may also receive vouchers for infant formula: each state contracts with one formula manufacturer such as Enfamil or Nestlé to provide discounted formula to WIC clients, and clients must use their vouchers for that contract brand unless they have a prescription stating that they have a medical need for a different formula. While WIC's limitations were restrictive, Lynne explained why she thought they were good for her family, saying, "You're already in the healthy products aisle. So it kind of [constrains] you. Instead of going down the chips and dip aisle, you want to go get vegetables." Sticking to the sections of the store where fresh dairy, meat, and produce are stored is a strategy known as "shopping the perimeter" and has been promoted by public health advocates as a way to eat more healthfully; shopping with WIC vouchers implicitly encouraged Lynne and others to adopt this strategy.[6]

Lynne and Vanessa were typical among low-income mothers in their appreciation for WIC's health advice. As part of the Food and Nutrition Service arm of the US Department of Agriculture, WIC has guidelines that reflect mainstream, government-endorsed positions on pregnancy health, nutrition, weight management, and breastfeeding. Local WIC offices, supervised by registered dietitians, were often housed in the same buildings as county public health services, and they worked with Medicaid to connect their low-income clients with medical care. As a result, clients' visits to WIC were integrated into their use of public health services more generally.

WIC's nutrition education program worked largely through the two complementary approaches Vanessa and Lynne cited. Counselors at WIC aimed to teach clients about healthy eating, informing them about the nutritional benefits and harms of different foods, using visual aids to illustrate portion size and food variety, and—when moms like Vanessa had difficulty getting children to eat healthfully—offering strategies for introducing nutritious foods. Diya shared one example of how she approached nutrition education: "We were teaching [clients] fifty percent of all grains should be whole grains. We're providing them with [vouchers for] whole grains. . . . Then sometimes I swap recipes with them, and I'm like 'Oh, have you tried this? I make an enchilada bake with the corn tortillas.' Instead of making enchiladas for an individual, for a family it's a lot harder. So just make a bake, and it's like lasagna, but with Mexican ingredients. [I talk about] using our foods that we provide and teaching them how they can incorporate that into healthy meal planning."

In this way, Diya and her colleagues in Florida tried to convey nutritional standards while making them feel achievable to low-income families that were often pressed for time. In California, the WIC program even published a cookbook of recipes that incorporated WIC-eligible foods, which local offices handed out free of charge to clients.

WIC then reinforced this education through the food voucher coupons it provided, guiding clients into the supermarket aisles where WIC-approved products could be purchased. As Lynne explained, hunting down WIC-eligible foods in the grocery store led her to the sections of the store she saw as "healthier" and away from junk food, disciplining her shopping practices even beyond what was covered by WIC.

Most WIC clients I interviewed voiced appreciation for the program. They believed that the health standards WIC promoted were essentially beneficial, and they generally saw the program's counselors as well intentioned and devoted to caring for mothers' and children's health. But not every mother followed WIC's recommendations. Some, like Jazmine Easton (Black, thirty-four, LL), found WIC's health tips difficult to follow: "[WIC told me] don't eat more fries, they're fattening, but I still did it of course! I tried to change, but it's hard to just say I ain't going to do this or eat that." Jazmine found the prohibition on fries too inflexible, making no provision for her own tastes. Others found it challenging but nonetheless aspired to follow WIC advice. May Campbell (Black, forty, LL), an Afro-Caribbean immigrant in Florida, added, "There's a lot of stuff I didn't really know, or I kind of did know but just wasn't interested in. But when it came down to my child, I had to step up my game." May was not interested in making permanent dietary changes for herself, but she tried to eat more vegetables when she was pregnant, believing that those investments would yield the greatest benefit to her children's long-term well-being.

Other mothers, especially mixed-class women with incomes low enough to qualify for WIC but who had higher levels of education, described WIC advice as "simple" and sought to do more. For example, Gita Potter (Asian, twenty-seven, HL), a California mother of one who had recently become pregnant again, explained, "It's stuff that I already know. I am not the kind of person who eats macaroni and cheese for every meal anyway. . . . I like to prepare healthy things anyway and have balanced meals just because I know that's better for our bodies. I can see how if I wasn't raised in a household where those things were taught that this might be really groundbreaking news. But it's really pretty simple stuff that I know about." Because she saw WIC's advice as good but "simple," Gita primarily valued the money she saved using WIC and followed her own, stricter beliefs when it came to her own reproductive body project. Gita rhetorically distanced herself from the type of person she imagined might have a harder time following WIC's advice, asserting that she was not the "kind of person" who might default to unhealthy eating ("macaroni and cheese for every meal") while suggesting that some people know less about good nutrition because of how they were raised.

Nicki Lindsay (white, thirty, HL) was a pastor's wife and stay-at-home mother of two living in Florida. Like Gita, she positioned herself as endorsing WIC advice while defining herself in contrast to other WIC recipients. Describing a roundtable discussion of breastfeeding at WIC she attended while pregnant, she explained,

> Some of the girls were not as interested, and I was kind of trying to encourage that breastfeeding is a good thing, and that it doesn't hurt after a while. That you get used to it, and it's so convenient. I guess I feel like [WIC] could have done a better job at encouraging them in that. It's tough, because the poor nutritionist feels like she's speaking to a wall. . . . But I thought it was good. I thought that some of the girls that were in there maybe came away with a different mindset, and maybe would consider breastfeeding, when maybe they wouldn't before that.

Nicki, who grew up middle-class and had a college degree, aligned herself ideologically with the WIC staff—viewing them as peers she could assist—rather than with her fellow WIC clients (whom she called "girls"). Like Gita, she worked to create a horizontal relationship with WIC staff as co-experts and rejected the position of knowledge recipient that many other WIC clients occupied. And, like Gita, she viewed WIC's health advice as well intentioned, if basic.

WIC clients came from a diverse range of backgrounds, with widely varying ages and levels of experience as parents. While some, like mixed-class Gita and Nicki, felt that WIC was not telling them anything they did not already know, others struggled to change their habits to better match the health norms WIC promoted. But all were fairly united in the belief that WIC staff members were trustworthy sources of advice and that the health standards WIC promoted were legitimate.

The same trust and personal relationships that facilitated low-income mothers' utilization of WIC advice also showed up, for some, in the relationships they built with physicians. Like WIC staff, physicians served as a source of authoritative knowledge about health and body-care standards; those who had an impact typically acknowledged clients' barriers to meeting those standards and worked with them to find solutions. Patrice Martin (Black, thirty-six, LL) explained what her relationship with her previous doctor had meant to her:

> She was the first doctor ever, in the history [of] every doctor I ever had, that gave me her cell number. . . . And she was even going to come out and do home visits with me, and when I went to the office she came and gave me a hug every day I came in there. When she left last year, I cried. I actually cried! . . . I bet she went out of state to work. The doctor I got now, she's a little bit younger, but they leave so darn quick, and I ain't going to get used to her because . . . she's going to Africa to work. So you know, you build up a relationship with these people and they be gone. But my other doctor, we had a pretty good, long relationship, and I cried when she left.

As a single mother raising four children on her own, Patrice poured her energies into her children and her work; despite concerns about her blood pressure and weight, she struggled to make time for herself. Her previous doctor, Patrice noted, "stayed on me about things," encouraging Patrice to share her concerns and checking up on her by phone. Patrice respected the new doctor's knowledge—even though she was "a little bit younger"—but, lacking the closeness and personal accountability of her relationship with her former doctor, she felt adrift when it came to taking concrete steps toward better health. Patrice's comment that doctors "leave so darn quick" also points to a problem faced by many of my low-income respondents, especially those living in rural or underresourced communities: shortages and high turnover rates among physicians made it harder to build the kind of relationships that many women found so critical for learning about and adopting healthful habits.[7]

In short, poor and working-class women I spoke to took medical and nutrition advice seriously. They tended to trust WIC staff and doctors, particularly those who appeared to genuinely care about building relationships with the women and their families. And they got most of their information about medical norms for their reproductive body projects through these relationships, using this information to inform their health practices and to verify the sometimes-conflicting advice they received from friends and family members.

### "I tend to take my physician's suggestions with a grain of salt": Middle- and Upper-Class Mothers Engaging with Health Expertise

Medical and scientific knowledge played an important role in middle- and upper-class mothers' reproductive body projects, too. These women tended to pursue the most up-to-date health and parenting practices, a sign of their moral devotion to healthism. Accordingly, they prioritized learning about scientific research on the benefits and harms of various approaches, and they used doctors' opinions and expert recommendations to justify the choices they made. But while poor and working-class women's access to health information often depended on the personal, vertical relationships they established with doctors and nutritionists, college-educated women were more likely to do extensive reading on their own and to treat medical professionals instrumentally: selected because they supported mothers' chosen approaches to health, providing skilled service, but not treated as the sole authorities on health.

For high-status women, doctors typically were one important source of information and support among many. Charlotte Moran, a biracial thirty-two-year-old living in California, told me that for questions about her daughter's health, she would first ask her own mother or her best friend, adding that "depending on what kind of question it was," she would definitely ask her daughter's doctor. Without pause, she rattled off a list of other sources: "There are websites that I look at regularly. Babycenter.com. Or books—Dr. Sears is my favorite. Also, I have a mom's group." Nadia Bernard (white, thirty-six, HH) added, "I finally have a general practitioner, and I really like her. So I would probably talk to her. She's on e-mail, which is amazing. I don't know if she always e-mails me back, but just knowing that she's said it's okay, and I have her e-mail address, is cool. . . . And then there's the Internet. I would google anything and everything! I like AskMoxie.com. She has a lot of mothering stuff on there, and her approach is pretty in line with mine." Both Charlotte and Nadia had solid, supportive relationships with their doctors that they could draw on if they needed health advice, but neither saw that relationship as sufficient for providing all of the information they might want. Instead, each wove together a support network comprised of horizontal relationships with family members and peers, medical professionals, and specialized references like parenting websites or books that reflected their personal tastes and priorities.

Middle- and upper-class women often arrived at their doctors' appointments with requests for specific tests or treatments that they had learned about online, and they checked advice from their medical providers against information they gleaned from parenting books, scientific journal articles, and recommendations from professional medical organizations. For example, when I asked Florida mother Rhea Weston (white, twenty-three, HH) whether she had a close relationship with her physician, she responded, "Sometimes we conflict on our opinions. . . . She said that there is no value in breastfeeding past a year and, you know, American Academy of Pediatrics and the World Health Organization both say that's really not true—there's a lot of benefits."

For breastfeeding support, Rhea instead turned to her local chapter of La Leche League (a national network of breastfeeding advocacy and support groups), where she learned about these benefits and used that information to inform her practice of extended breastfeeding with her thirteen-month-old son. Similarly, Jessie Wozniak, a thirty-one-year-old white Florida mother, told me that while she loved her son's pediatrician, "If something just doesn't sit right or I'm curious, I look it up online or go to a resource."

The health resources women cited in our interviews together frequently included a mixture of print and online media: books from the *What to Expect When You're Expecting* series and Dr. Sears's *Baby Book* were the most popular; websites like BabyCenter.com and the local parenting listservs in each of the two areas where I conducted interviews were also frequently mentioned, as were print periodicals like *Parents* magazine. And numerous other respondents cited Internet searches, academic journal articles, and favorite blogs as primary sources for information. Critically, nearly all mentions of websites, books, and magazines came from middle- and mixed-class women; a handful of working-class women cited books from the bestselling *What to Expect* series, but otherwise, low-income women seemed to be googling health issues in response to acute issues that came up, rather than having books or websites that they read regularly as part of a day-to-day habit of consuming health advice.

Another widespread pattern was that many high-status respondents either worked as health professionals or had close friends and family members who did; others were highly educated professionals who had access to leading scientific journals like *Pediatrics* or the *Journal of the American Medical Association* through institutional subscriptions. For example, Hillary Kirk (white, twenty-six, HH) was a law student in Florida who explained, "I'm a researcher, so [I go to the] Internet. . . . I search for hours, until I find a vast amount of evidence to support whatever it is." Other mothers, like Lucy Wolff (white, thirty-three, HH), noted the importance of checking one's Internet sources: "MayoClinic.com and stuff like that is a little more reputable than 'myhealthblog.com'!" And MacKenzie Gervais (white, thirty, HH) added, "I don't trust sites like Wikipedia. . . . [I look at] WebMD or some of the medical sites. And I prefer to get it from more than one place, because at the end of the day, everything is written by a human being and there is going to be a bias, whether you like it or not." In this way, MacKenzie and other mothers sought to demonstrate their expertise at gathering information and evaluating sources.

Amanda Katz (white, thirty, HH), a registered nurse living in Florida, used her institutional access to look up academic resources. She explained, "Google Health is good. I usually use the Google Scholar search engine if I'm looking for something more scholarly and specific."

I asked Amanda how being a healthcare provider had affected her approaches to caring for her own health or her son's, and her response surprised me: "I tend to take my physician's suggestions with a grain of salt. They're people just like anyone else. If you've worked with physicians, [you know] they put their pants on one leg at a time, take a poop every day. . . . I just feel like even though you want the scientific basis for [making health decisions] it's not always going to happen; a lot of things are done by tradition."

Interestingly, Amanda's intimate knowledge of medicine—as a provider and through her professional interactions with doctors—had made her skeptical of medical recommendations; she valued evidence-based medicine when the evidence was available, but she was also acutely aware that doctors were human beings—people who "take a poop every day," just like everyone else—who sometimes based their guidance on tradition, not evidence. Lori Kent (white, twenty-nine, HH), who was working on her PhD in chemistry, said, "We have a friend who is a doctor, so sometimes when we have true medical questions, we'll just call him up and ask him." Recently, however, she had hassled her doctor friend while she was, in her words, "a little bit inebriated": "I told him that medicine was voodoo science. And while I don't completely believe that, I think that sometimes it's true. Just the way that their research is completely different than the way that I think of research in chemistry."

For Amanda and Lori, as for many other middle- and upper-class mothers, social closeness to doctors and other medical professionals as peers and colleagues—rather than as distant authority figures—made them feel comfortable challenging medical authority when it came to decisions about their family's health. Annette Lareau describes this comfort as a distinctive feature of middle-class *entitlement*, in which class-privileged parents ask health providers probing questions, push for customized care, and teach their children to do the same. Lareau argues that when middle-class parents model this interactional style (as opposed to the more deferential working-class style), their "children discover that their own opinions are valued by others, that their ideas are considered interesting and important," and they develop a sense of entitlement to attentive, personal care from high-status adults.[8]

Middle- and upper-class women's challenges to doctors did not mean that they were anti-science or anti-medicine; rather, they leveraged evidence from both conventional medical research and other sources to get more individualized care (supporting their personal health goals and values) and to resist unwanted medicalization of their bodies. For example, Britta Larson (white, thirty-nine, HH) challenged her doctor's recommendation that she lose weight during pregnancy due to her relatively high body mass index (BMI); she contended that "body mass index is bullshit, honestly," and then outlined to her doctor what she was already doing to care for her health through rigorous exercise. She concluded, "I understand what you're doing here [with the BMI standards], but I think that this is aimed at a different group of people who happen to be the same size as me and have nothing to do with me." With this statement, Britta rejected the one-size-fits-all model of care dictated by the BMI guidelines, instead pushing her doctor to look at her body holistically by considering her activity level and other measures of health. Britta's confrontation with her doctor offers a sharp contrast to the approaches that low-income mothers like Jazmine Easton took: when Jazmine found WIC's dietary guidelines too restrictive, she simply did not follow them; when Britta experienced similar one-size-fits-all health recommendations, she felt empowered to challenge her healthcare provider and demand more personalized care.

Lucy Wolff (white, thirty-three, HH), currently pregnant with her first child, told me why she had opted to work with a midwife instead of an obstetrician: "I didn't want unnecessary medical interventions. I didn't want my pregnancy and birth being treated as sort of a disease, I guess. And I had read that with a midwife you're less likely to have unwanted cesareans, unwanted episiotomies, and other interventions."

Numerous middle- and upper-class women voiced similar sentiments, preferring to work with midwives and doulas, to try for unmedicated or minimally medicated labor, or even to attempt home birth, all to avoid what they saw as excessive medical surveillance. A small minority were openly antagonistic toward medical professionals, but most viewed doctors and medicine as occupying an important, if circumscribed position: providing personalized guidance—balanced out by women's own research and priorities—for the care of mothers' and children's health.

## Working with—and against—Grandmothers

While doctors, public health officials, and popular or scientific health publications offered women guidance according to medical norms for the body, a second major source of information and support came from women's own mothers: their children's grandmothers. Most women's models for raising children came from their own experiences of being mothered—even if, as in some cases, they defined their parenting in opposition to their mothers' approaches. And women's mothers, especially those who lived nearby, were often a source of everyday, hands-on support in caring for babies; even when such grandmothers held health and body-care values that conflicted with current medical recommendations, those who saw their daughters and grandchildren regularly tended to exert a powerful influence on women's reproductive body projects.

### *"She's always there to help me": Poor and Working-Class Mothers and Grandmothers*

Among poor and working-class women I spoke to, grandmothers provided some of the most immediate, consistent support and advice. Florida mother Kathryn Schmidt (white, twenty-four, LL) offered an example of how such arrangements came about. Kathryn had gotten pregnant shortly after she began dating her boyfriend, Mike. Despite the newness of their relationship, Mike and Kathryn decided to continue the pregnancy and, when Mike moved to Michigan for work, they planned that she would follow him once the baby was born. This plan unraveled when Mike broke up with Kathryn via text message five months into her pregnancy. During the six months that had passed since the birth of their son, Kayden, Mike would occasionally reach out with an offer to reconcile or be involved in Kayden's life, but these gestures were stressful and upsetting to Kathryn; Mike frequently misspelled Kayden's name and, on more than one occasion, texted from his new girlfriend's phone. Given Mike's absence and unpredictability (or, as Kathryn put it, "being an idiot"), Kathryn turned to her mother for support. "We moved back in with my mom when Mike left so I wouldn't have to get my own place. . . . Now, I'm just trying to get back on my feet." When I asked her if her mother helped her out, she responded,

"Yeah. She'll come home, and if he's been fussy or something she'll take him and help calm him down."

As I spoke to Kathryn, her mother—holding Kayden—popped in to suggest that it might be time for a feeding; the two women negotiated who would handle the feeding with a familiarity born of living together and sharing childcare duties over the previous six months. Afterward, Kathryn noted that her mother not only cared for Kayden but supported Kathryn as well, encouraging her to get out of the house and attend fitness classes at the local county health department.

Of the twenty-six poor and working-class mothers I interviewed, half (thirteen) lived with extended family members, most often, like Kathryn, with their own mothers and siblings. Seventeen were unmarried (nine had boyfriends, eight were single). Women who lived with their mothers (whom I will refer to as "grandmothers" as shorthand) often relied on these arrangements to provide flexible, free childcare and/or financial support. Such was the case for Kathryn, whose mother helped give her an occasional break from the stress of managing a needy infant as well as providing a place to live, rent free. Many respondents also described these living arrangements as helpful for pooling resources: mothers of young children brought food into the household through their WIC benefits (which are permitted to be shared with any family member living in the home); various household members contributed cash via paid work, child support payments, and welfare benefits; and household members who did not work for pay—usually women such as my respondents, their mothers, or their sisters—looked after the children of those who did.

Given these arrangements, when I asked respondents to whom they would turn for health advice, many poor and working-class women responded as Kathryn did: "[My mom] is the first person I'd go to if I need anything. If I had a question, she's the first person I'd go to." Kathryn and others saw their mothers as seasoned parents who had practical, hands-on knowledge about how to take care of a child. Additionally, they trusted that their mothers would have their children's best interests at heart. Rosa Acosta (Latina, nineteen, LL) explained how her mother stepped in when Rosa became pregnant the previous year. "She always gives me good advice and whenever I need something, she's always there to help me. . . . I didn't use to eat a lot of beans, but my mom said that was good because that had iron. So, I started eating beans and a little bit more vegetables than I ate before. It was a little bit hard because sometimes I ate stuff that I really didn't like. But you know, my mom told me if I wanted a healthy baby, I had to make a change."

Rosa's close-knit, Catholic, immigrant family was disappointed that Rosa had become pregnant and dropped out of high school during her senior year. Still, Rosa's parents supported her and her daughter, providing financially so that Rosa could stay home to breastfeed and work toward her GED. At the same time, they made sure Rosa met her responsibilities as a mother, adopting a "tough love" approach that Rosa found both helpful and, at times, isolating. When I visited Rosa at her parents' home for our interview, she was folding laundry and keeping an eye on her napping seven-month-old; I asked her if she ever got a break to spend time with her friends and she responded, "My parents . . . tell me that it doesn't look right if I go out anymore because I already have a daughter, and I should stay home with her." For Rosa, accessing her parents' support meant accepting their judgment as well; all were in unspoken agreement that Rosa's financial dependence gave her parents the right to comment on her choices. In this period, which the scholarly literature terms "emerging adulthood" (roughly ages eighteen to twenty-five), it is common for young people to cohabit with or otherwise financially rely on their parents to make the transition to full adulthood, working toward academic attainment, paid employment, independent living, and more. But while this sustained parental support can help set young people up for better outcomes in the long term, it also brings the potential for conflict as parents and their adult children renegotiate their roles and relationships to one another.[9]

Many poor and working-class mothers' relationships with their own mothers—whether or not they lived in the same household—were characterized by this mixture of closeness, dependency, and control. Some women, like Rosa, followed their mothers' advice; others resented it. May Campbell's current caregiving responsibilities included both her two youngest children and her oldest son's baby daughter, her first grandchild. She recalled the advice she had received from her mother when she was a young parent, now revisiting it from her new perspective as a grandmother herself. "My mama was trying to tell me what to do, but I just didn't feel like I should have been breastfeeding anyway. . . .

She's a mom, they know best, but me? No, I wasn't listening. She knew what was best for me, but me, growing up, a teenager, I don't want to hear nothing. I think I know it all already."

Kiara Jefferson (Black, twenty, LL), a Florida mother of one child who was pregnant with her second, was similarly ambivalent about receiving help from her mother. At the time I interviewed her, Kiara was sitting on the porch of her mother's home, where she lived with her three-year-old daughter, her mother, her brother, and four of her nieces and nephews. As we spoke, the sounds of the five young children playing and shrieking echoed in the house. Kiara sighed, telling me about her eagerness to find an apartment of her own: "[My] baby daddy . . . he say he going to be there, but he not showing me [by] being here now, so I figure when the baby due he ain't gonna be here." I asked, "So you figure you're going to be doing this on your own?" She responded, "Yeah, or I'll ask my mom to help again. That's another thing I don't want to do, is ask for help. I don't want to keep asking her. That's why I want to get out on my own, so I can learn or get more experience as a mom."

Both May and Kiara described the difficult position many poor and working-class mothers found themselves in when, particularly as teenagers, they became parents. With a median age of twenty-one when they had their first child, poor and working-class women in my study tended to have little separation between being children and having children of their own. On one hand, this meant that they often still lived with or near their families of origin, making it much easier to share childcare with their families. On the other hand, many women like May and Kiara described the tension these close ties entailed: parent-child relationships are usually structured in a vertical hierarchy, and adult daughters living with their mothers often struggled to establish their own adulthood, bodily autonomy, and authority as mothers in their own right. Only years later could May admit that "[my mother] knew what was best for me, but me, growing up, a teenager, I don't want to hear nothing. I think I know it all already."

Not all women in this group appreciated their mothers' support, whether in the present or retrospectively. Some, such as Gaby Romero (Latina, twenty-nine, LL), described their mothers as "old-fashioned" and clashed with them over recommendations that were at odds with doctors' advice; others, like Nicole Johnson (Black, twenty-two, LL), were estranged from their mothers and received no help at all. Nonetheless, second only to medical providers, poor and working-class women's mothers were the most consistently cited sources of positive advice and support.

### "It's a lot harder to talk to someone in your mother's generation": Middle- and Upper-Class Mothers and Grandmothers

In contrast, middle- and upper-class women were much more likely to highlight differences of opinion they had with their own mothers. Stephanie Brewer (white, thirty-two, HH) told me how, living in the San Francisco Bay Area, she was the first woman in her group of friends to have a baby (at age twenty-eight). As a result, she had few peers with whom to discuss the bodily experiences that pregnancy brought. She said, "I just knew no one who had had a baby in thirty years! There's all these common experiences, every woman goes through it. But it's a lot harder to talk to someone in your mother's generation about the changes that are going on than it is to talk to somebody your own generation." Stephanie, like many other high-status mothers, emphasized the gulf of time separating her entry into motherhood from that of her own mother. Stephanie and her peers were, on average, thirty-one years old at the time they had their first child, mirroring nationwide trends among women with bachelor's degrees or higher.[10] As a result, the mothers of women in this class were further removed from their own childbearing years than those in the poor and working-class group. Middle- and upper-class mothers were, therefore, more likely to face different social norms and medical advice than their own mothers had received than were poor and working-class women. Many grandmothers in this group had their babies at a time when breastfeeding was less common. Joan Zimmerman (white, thirty-eight, HH), who had difficulty establishing a breastfeeding relationship with her first-born, recounted her mother-in-law's unhelpful advice about this: "She once said to me while I was struggling with Simon in the hospital, 'It was a lot easier, the way I did it,' which was bottle feeding. I have never wanted to punch an old lady before, but I wanted to punch her."

Not all middle- and upper-class mothers had such heated reactions to advice from their mothers and mothers-in-law, but many expressed frustration and discomfort with the suggestions they gave. Amy Chen (Asian, thirty-five, HH) told me that she preferred friends' advice to her own mother's, saying, "[I would ask] a lot of my girlfriends. They are most all moms by now. I don't talk to my mom as much, because she comes from a very different background and lifestyle." When I asked her to explain, she told me her mother believed in using traditional Chinese herbal and homeopathic medicines, while Amy—married to a white physician—preferred Western medicine.

Many other middle-class mothers described a similar phenomenon, but in reverse: European American grandmothers favored Western medicine, while their adult daughters sought out alternative and holistic medicine. Emily Fischer (white, thirty-one, HH), for example, disapproved of what she perceived to be her mother's overreliance on Western pharmaceuticals: "I don't want to end up like my mom. She's on a million medications. And her first reaction when I'll complain about something is, 'Oh, you should take such-and-such a pill.' Well, [sighing] I don't like that to be my first line of defense. So when I had some major health problems four years ago, she kept trying to get me on medication. 'Oh, well this helped so-and-so. And this one helped so-and-so.' And I was like, 'You know what? I think I'm going to try acupuncture.'"

As Amy's and Emily's stories show, middle-class women and their mothers' disagreements often differed in substance but shared a dynamic in which daughters did not perceive their mothers to be reliable, legitimate sources of knowledge about health and bodies. They frequently rejected traditional wisdom, instead seeking advice from peers and expert sources (such as doctors or medical research) in their quest to optimize their reproductive body projects.

Middle- and upper-class mothers' ambivalence about their mothers' support was due to more than just coming of age in an era with different health norms. These women's eschewal of their mothers' advice was made possible by the conditions of their lives. By the time they became mothers, most of the high-status women I spoke with had moved beyond "emerging adulthood" and established independent careers and households: all lived with their husbands and children, and only one—Lori Kent—resided with a member of her extended family at the time of our interview (Lori's mother had come to stay for the month after Lori's daughter was born, but she was not a permanent member of the household).

Women's geographic mobility was also a factor in keeping distance between women and their mothers: these women often lived hundreds or thousands of miles from family members. Indeed, multiple studies have found that higher education and higher socioeconomic status increase geographic mobility, and these trends were reflected in the stories of the women I interviewed.[11] According to many of the middle- and upper-class women I spoke to, maintaining emotional and geographic space from their mothers was important for their own well-being. Hillary Kirk (white, twenty-six, HH) explained how her strained relationship with her mother often centered around body issues: "I always thought my body was fine until I got to my teenage [years], and then my mom started to think about diets and stuff. I was tiny. . . . I was a horseback rider, so I did lots of events at the national and state level. I was really athletic, but still my mom needed to have me on a diet."

When Hillary applied to college, she made a point of getting some distance between herself and her mother, saying, "I went as far away from [my home state of] Michigan as I could get, really. I would have gone to California, but I didn't get into a school there." Hillary's mother continued to make disparaging comments about Hillary's body when they would see each other, especially after Hillary gained weight during her first year of college, but the distance between them made it easier for Hillary to shut her mother out. Later, when Hillary was pregnant and living in Florida, she recounted that her mother was still "big into commanding me to do things. . . . You need to eat this way or that way." In response, she said, "You try to block it out."

Like Hillary, Suzanne Walsh (white, thirty-five, HH) had a complicated relationship with her mother and her own body image. Suzanne disclosed that she struggled with anorexia and bulimia in her teens and twenties, a result, she believed, of a childhood spent watching her mother trying to stay thin through fasting and intensive exercise. As Suzanne recovered—starting to menstruate again and, eventually, getting pregnant—she wrestled with what closeness to her mother might cost her: "I've always struggled with eating disorder stuff. So part of my anger toward my mom was that I'd been so hyperconscious of my own road to recovery and my own process. . . . And my mom is very holier-than-thou about food and nutrition. . . . Being around her is very hard for me."

From both Suzanne's and Hillary's stories, it becomes clear that high-status women's widespread ambivalence about (and in some cases, outright rejection of) their mothers' advice is not only about their being unreliable sources of knowledge. Rather, like several low-income women cited earlier, these women frequently pushed back on their mothers in an effort to establish boundaries and autonomy: to escape the vertical relationships they had to their mothers as children. The difference was that, with greater financial independence and geographic distance, middle- and upper-class women had greater means with which to hold those boundaries firm.

## Peers as Positive and Negative References

The third major source of support that many women named was their peers: chosen communities with whom women could find solidarity, affirmation, and identity. Advice from older generations and medical providers to mothers tends to be unidirectional: handed down from people who have more experience as mothers and/or more expert credentials in health. In contrast, peer relationships offer mothers the chance to participate in a more equitable give and take of knowledge. Respondents who saw their peers as having strong health and body-care values and expertise—usually middle- and upper-class mothers—were particularly invested in building strong peer support networks; those who aspired toward upward mobility, on the other hand, tended to discount the value of what peers from their class of origin could offer them.

### "The moms I'm friends with coincide with the lifestyle I like": Middle- and Upper-Class Mothers and Peers

Higher-status women tended to discount their own mothers' perspectives, but they were much more enthusiastic about seeking—and giving—advice within peer groups made up of their contemporaries. Beyond all other sources of advice and support, middle- and upper-class women in my study most frequently turned to their peers: other mothers who tended to be of comparable age, education, and class background. Many women emphasized the importance of having friends and confidantes who shared compatible parenting approaches and value systems to one's own. I asked Florida mother MacKenzie Gervais (white, thirty, HH) to describe whom she would go to for advice about health issues, and she responded, "I put stock in what a lot of my friends have to say. A lot of us have small kids around the same age. . . . So I think most of my friends have healthy lifestyles I would trust." Likewise, Charlotte Moran (biracial, thirty-two, HH) explained to me that she would most trust her friend Aileen for advice about health issues, because "we have the same approach to eating and to life. So I would ask her, probably expecting to get back an answer that I would already have come up with." I inquired why that would be important to her, and Charlotte said, "To confirm what I was thinking. Sometimes I bounce things off her, hoping to hear what I already think. And when I don't, it makes me rethink what I was thinking."

For Charlotte, constructive criticism or disagreement with her chosen reproductive body project would only be welcome from someone with essentially similar values—someone whom she could trust to offer advice that supported, rather than undermined, her personal health goals. Drawn-out discussions of health and body choices were important to many highly educated mothers, a way to establish their health expertise and their status as morally good, risk-avoidant mothers (themes that will be explored in subsequent chapters). But these discussions could happen only in a context where the participants could build on a base of shared knowledge and values. Bree Turner (white, thirty-three, HH) explained how important these factors were when choosing her friends: "I have a lot of good girlfriends, a good social network of moms. They are right in it with me. They are not super athletes, but we're good athletes. We're strong. We've come a long way. A lot of them have had two kids or three kids. We value identity outside of being a mom."

Thus, even while Bree sought out friends who shared the experience of being mothers, she emphasized the importance of other aspects of identity besides motherhood. Similarly, Amy Chen told me that she felt particularly drawn to friends who valued the active, exercise-intensive lifestyle she prioritized. She described this orientation to her body, saying, "I always took care of my body, so I never wanted to let myself go, for any reason. Some people do; I just didn't want to. It was something I believed in." She continued, "The moms that I try to keep friends with coincide with the lifestyle that I like." For Amy, finding friends who shared her attitudes toward food, exercise, health, and self-control was a way of bolstering her own commitment to not "letting herself go" following childbirth, and to maintaining a consistent sense of self-identity.

For some women, finding these like-minded peers to support their decisions and reinforce their sense of self happened easily, as when multiple friends in a social circle became pregnant around the same time. For others, such networks did not exist, so they instead sought to build or join intentional communities: "mommy groups." Not all peer networks consisted of equally strong ties. At minimum, most middle- and upper-class women in my study subscribed to one or more mothering websites or electronic listservs, where they could post questions on a range of topics or provide answers to other women's queries. Participation in such diffuse networks offered mothers the benefit of a wide range of opinions and recommendations; at the same time, many women took part in those conversations by "lurking," reading other members' comments but never offering their own input. Bree spoke appreciatively about the group she belonged to: "I feel like I'm lucky to have that closeness, and people are in the same boat, so we can commiserate and talk." Mixed-class Louise Peralta (white, thirty-six, LH) added, "When I lay [my daughter] down to change her diaper, she's kicking at me. She's slapping at me, trying to hit me. And I don't know what to do. . . . I actually posed a question about it on [my local mothering listserv]. 'Is this normal? What can I do?' See if anybody can help me." But while Louise was a frequent visitor to the group's electronic message board and a consumer of the advice she found there, a recent experience had demonstrated to her the limits of the closeness this online community could provide. A few months before I interviewed her, Louise decided to take her children to an Easter egg hunt sponsored by the group.

> We went to one of their events at Easter time this year. . . . And basically, everybody ignored us. . . . It was a waste of our time, and I don't want my daughters to feel like they're being shunned, you know? Maybe if we spent more time with these people, they would be a little warmer. But it seemed like they already kind of knew each other and we were the new people and [their attitude was] "We don't want to know you." Nobody made an effort to know us. Nobody said hi or anything, so we just said, "Forget it. We're not going to do that."

Louise tied her feelings around this event to similar experiences she had had as a child, when her rural, farming background set her apart from her town-dwelling classmates (an association suggesting that Louise sensed that her shunning might be partially class based). For Louise, finding herself and her children snubbed at the event was a rude awakening, given the intimate details and support that these same women shared online. Indeed, other women noted to me that what made online support groups work was, precisely, their anonymity; the intimacy that anonymity facilitated did not necessarily translate well into in-person familiarity.

Many other women found peer reference groups by joining in-person activities geared toward new and expectant mothers, such as prenatal yoga classes and breastfeeding support groups like La Leche League. In some cases, women found mommy groups through the hospital where they delivered; Florida mothers Cass Blackwell and Emily Fischer, whom I interviewed together, had met and become friends through a postpartum depression support group organized by their medical provider. Still other women formed communities once they enrolled their children in daycare together or joined postpartum exercise groups. What made many of these activity-based communities particularly strong was that they enabled women to connect on the basis of shared values, interests, and identities—and shared reproductive body projects—beyond simply being mothers. In other words, not just any group of mothers would do as a source of support; women sought out particular groups that validated their personal ideals and identities, including—but not limited to—motherhood. As Bree noted, she had cultivated friendships with women who "value identity outside of being a mom."

There were, however, down sides to the homogeneity and homegrown health expertise that middle- and upper-class women's peer support networks offered. In addition to the exclusionary dynamics that Louise witnessed, these groups had the ability to circulate unhelpful—or even harmful—health advice, as Amy Chen described: "When I joined a mommy group here, not only was there culture shock, being in California—it's so different from being in Boston—but the biggest difference, I thought, was about vaccinations. . . . A lot of moms had strong opinions [against childhood vaccines] and it was so hard for me not to be rude. Like, 'Okay, maybe it's just a West Coast thing.' All my friends [back in Boston] had their kids vaccinated. Why wouldn't they? You're doing a disservice to your child by not giving them the vaccination."

Accustomed to questioning medical authority and "doing their own research," several members of Amy's new social circle insisted on delaying or avoiding vaccines for their children, basing their decisions on scientifically unsupported fears of vaccine injuries; they shared these views widely within online and in-person social networks. The effects of these discourses—most common among middle- and upper-class parents—were significant: during the early 2000s, California saw large increases in the number of parents claiming "personal belief exemptions" (PBEs) to vaccine mandates for entering public school.[12] Following a large measles outbreak—tied to transmission among unvaccinated people at Disneyland—in 2014–2015, a few years after I spoke to Amy, California passed legislation eliminating new PBE petitions; in 2019, the state passed a second bill aimed at limiting the criteria for medical exemptions to vaccination requirements.[13]

In Florida, too, class-privileged women like Masha Begovic (white, thirty-four, HH) and Hillary Kirk (white, twenty-six, HH), as well as mixed-class, college-educated Noura Berry (white, twenty-three, LH), resisted vaccinating their children on the basis of their distrust of medical authority and their confidence in their own health expertise. Masha, who had recently moved to Florida from California, explained her views thus:

> They say if you have [the vaccine] and then you do get chickenpox later it should be a milder case. But who is going to tell me that? I haven't seen it. When did it start? I don't know people who got [the shots] when they were young, so I don't know how the case will be. Is it going to be as mild as they say it will? I don't know. So I would prefer if [my children] got chickenpox as soon as possible. Get it over with so I won't have to worry about revaccinations. . . . But you tell that to a doctor and they get so arrogant about it. "Absolutely not! You have to get the vaccine." . . . They try to convince you and they don't even discuss other options with you. They give you that attitude. So I stopped arguing, because I'm not stupid and I'm definitely not uneducated. And I'm doing my research, and that's why I'm arguing with them.

Masha described what her "research" looked like: "I rely on Google. And my friends, especially the ones from California, or the ones here with degrees. I'm scanning the friends I know here; anybody who has a master's or PhD will have done some Google checking and probably will be a breastfeeding mom and buying organic food."

Illustrating Jennifer Reich's finding that vaccine skepticism is most common among middle- and upper-class parents,[14] Masha claimed the authority to reject doctors' advice due to her belief in her own expertise ("I'm doing my research," "I'm not uneducated") and to the reinforcement she got for her views from similarly situated, class-privileged women ("friends from California" and "anybody who has a master's or PhD"). Among middle- and upper-class women I interviewed, similar dynamics arose around other health and body topics such as diet and infant feeding: a sense of personal expertise, coupled with support from trusted peers, could furnish women with a sense of empowerment, but it could also become a breeding ground for misinformation that was, at best, medically unhelpful and, at worst, harmful.

In sum, while middle- and upper-class women did not join formal, government-sponsored discussions on health (such as the ones low-income women in WIC were required to attend), they nevertheless sought out and participated in informal institutions in the form of mommy groups. Such groups enabled mothers to connect with similarly situated peers who shared their values and priorities for health and childrearing. Relationships within these groups tended to be horizontal, rather than vertical: with no built-in hierarchies due to generation (as exist between mothers and daughters) or professional expertise (as in the relationship between doctors and patients), middle- and upper-class mothers could enjoy having the chance to both give and receive advice with their peers. Additionally, given that many groups were based in particular neighborhoods and communities, that they required participants to have leisure time, and that some cost money to join, participants tended to share class and racial homogeneity. The groups offered emotional support and norm reinforcement, disciplining and bolstering middle- and upper-class women's ongoing commitment to shared health and body values. Such shared health values, however, did not always translate into beneficial health practices and outcomes.

### "They're nobody I would try to follow": Low-Income Mothers and Peers

In contrast, poor and working-class women in my study were much less likely to cite peers as useful sources of support and knowledge about health and parenting. Those who did turn to peers tended to speak about the meanings of these ties in different terms than did higher-status mothers, emphasizing one-on-one relationships over groups, and prioritizing emotional closeness and reliability over specialized knowledge and shared health values. Furthermore, low-income women's reliance on peer support appeared to be racialized: poor and working-class white women were somewhat more likely to rely on peers, while Black and Latina mothers tended to describe their peers as unreliable sources of information and poor role models.

As noted above, so-called mommy groups tended to attract women from similar neighborhoods, educational backgrounds, and interests—all of which promote class homogeneity in the group (specifically, middle-to-upper-class identity). The experiences of the few mixed-class women who participated in these groups highlight this dynamic. As described earlier, Louise Peralta had grown up working class but was more economically middle class at the time I interviewed her; when she tried to attend an in-person meet-up for mothers and children in her area, she experienced a subtle sense of misfit that seemed to be a product of her class-mismatched cultural capital. Cass Blackwell (white, thirty-three, LH), who had experienced upward mobility similar to Louise's, fared a little better in her group. I interviewed Cass alongside one of the other members of her postpartum support group, Emily Fischer (white, twenty-six, HH). Each woman took turns answering my questions, but an interesting dynamic developed between them. While Cass was older than Emily—and both were first-time parents—Emily was much more confident in her answers to my questions about health and body-care choices. Both women's babies were teething, and I asked how they were dealing with their babies' pain and fussiness. Emily explained that her approach was to ask, "What other things can I try before I drug her up?" and then try swaddling or bouncing before resorting to infant Tylenol. Cass echoed Emily's reservations about medication and added, "As soon as we got home from the hospital, we forgot about the swaddling, so that's always the last thing that we come to. But [my daughter's] not big on the swaddling at this point anymore, 'cause her arms are constantly flailing. But we try the Hyland's teething tablets, which is homeopathic."

Cass began to explain how the tablets worked when Emily interrupted, "Those were just recalled!" "All of them?" asked Cass. "Yeah, I think so," Emily responded. Cass looked sheepish and immediately started to backpedal on her use of the tablets, saying, "Well, it's just a sugar tablet type thing, and it doesn't really do much for her anyway when we did try it. So we're pretty much just at Tylenol and loving comfort." At the time I interviewed Emily and Cass, the Hyland's recall was fairly recent; Emily's interjection was probably meant in the spirit of sharing health information, but it served to position Emily as the more knowledgeable of the two, putting Cass on the spot. Indeed, throughout their interview Cass frequently modified her answers to better agree with Emily's strongly stated positions. Although they were technically peers, Cass and Emily's relationship contained a vertical element, perhaps a relic of Cass's working-class origins. Like Louise, Cass was something of an outsider in the social circles she now frequented; unlike Louise, she seemed able to manage that tension, deferring to Emily's expertise while trying to keep up.

Few low-income mothers took part in mommy groups or other formal peer networks. Some, however, did rely on individual friends or same-age family members. Utilization of peer-to-peer relationships for support varied by race and ethnicity. Fewer than half of the twenty-six poor and working-class women I interviewed said that their peers were a positive source of health information or support, but of those who did, almost all were white (seven out of ten white working-class mothers). Only one of four Latina mothers—Mercedes—cited a friend's support as being helpful for her health and body-care goals, and only two out of twelve Black mothers did so. In contrast, twelve of the twenty-six low-income women I spoke to specifically called out their peers as being unhelpful when it came to health and body-care issues, and several more neglected to mention friends or same-aged mothers when I asked them to list the people in their lives whom they might ask for support. Mothers who explicitly described their peers as unhelpful when it came to health and body care were predominantly women of color: more than half (seven out of twelve) of Black mothers and three of four Latina respondents, compared to a minority (two out of ten) of white women. While these numbers are small overall—and thus we should be conservative about drawing too many conclusions from them—they are, at least, suggestive of racialized patterns in mothers' reliance on peer support.

Poor and working-class women in my study tended to be younger—by about ten years, on average—than middle- and upper-class women I interviewed. Yet when these young women described the minimal support they got from peers, it was not due to a lack of peers who had children. Shawna Blanchard (Black, twenty-two, LL), currently pregnant with her first child, explained that when it came to her health, she would go to "nobody young. I look up to someone that's older who had more experience." She added, "I'm actually the last of my friends to be pregnant. Everybody has a baby. They really don't have nothing to say, I guess, because we all still young and we still dealing with both working and trying to do school too. They really don't have nothing to say. They not nobody that I would try to follow. Everybody kind of is in their own world . . . but ain't nobody really saving money, going to school, and working. They not really all on a good level."

Because of their youth, Shawna did not see her peers as good models to emulate as she looked toward the responsibilities of motherhood. Like her, they were trying to get their lives together, balancing work and school (though, in Shawna's eyes, not always very successfully). Interestingly, Shawna also answered my question about caring for her child's health and body by talking about saving money and going to school, suggesting that for her, promoting her baby's well-being was, first and foremost, tied to long-term financial stability.

California mother Nicole Johnson (Black, twenty-two, LL) voiced similar sentiments about her peers when I spoke to her. Nicole was estranged from her own mother, a habitual drug user whose addiction had left her unable to care for Nicole and her siblings. Nicole had dropped out of school at age fourteen to work and support her younger brother and sister, and all three children had spent time in the foster care system. When Nicole got pregnant at sixteen, she transferred to a residential program for at-risk teens to earn her high school diploma. There, she shared an apartment with several other pregnant girls in the program, some of whom she referred to as her "cousins."[15] I commented on the serendipity of this timing, and I asked whether, since Nicole's mother was out of the picture, Nicole enjoyed having same-age kin to talk to. Nicole laughed and responded,

> No, I didn't even like to be around them like that. Everyone else had their second kid. I was the only one that didn't have another child [and] I was the only one working. I would never have another child if I'm not ready . . . and then they all had another kid and I was like, "You just can't keep having kids when you can't even afford a loaf of bread." . . . We all went our own distance away from each other because I got to keep going to school. Education is the biggest thing I have to worry [about] in order to pay for me and my kid. I was on a more independent road than everyone else.

Nicole, like Shawna, considered many of her peers to be bad role models because she believed they did not share her commitment to education and hard work. Nicole's biography certainly provided evidence of this commitment: while she continued to receive WIC benefits for help buying groceries, she had also completed her high school education and was currently pursuing a bachelor's degree in education while working full-time. In some ways, Nicole's and Shawna's choices about whom to associate with—and whom to avoid—were similar to the values-driven rationales given by upper-middle-class women like Amy Chen, who stated, "The moms that I try to keep friends with coincide with the lifestyle that I like." In other ways, racialized class differences affected the substance of Nicole's and Shawna's values and affiliations. Whereas many middle- and upper-class women sought out friends who shared their specific childcare philosophies or exercise and nutrition practices, Nicole's and Shawna's priorities—like those of many Black and Latina women from low-income backgrounds—centered more on financial stability and upward mobility. Furthermore, while higher-class women typically cited these values as positive drivers of friendship—strengthening their bonds to mothers who shared their priorities—poor and working-class women like Nicole and Shawna spoke more consistently in the negative, using their values to explain why they avoided or cut ties with certain peers.

Very few LL women used the language of shared health and parenting values to describe the friends they chose. Instead, those who cited their friends as sources of support for their reproductive body projects—white women, for the most part—prioritized loyalty and dependability over health expertise: they could talk to these friends about body issues because they could talk to them about anything.

For example, Sarah Evans (white, twenty-one, LL) listed her mother and her WIC nutritionist as primary sources of advice about health and body issues. Then she added, "My best friend would just let me know that whatever I should do with my body, in a good way, she'd give me 100 percent support. If I felt like I need to lose ten pounds, exercise, eat right, [she'd tell me to] do what I have to do to get it off." Likewise, Mercedes Diaz (Latina, nineteen, LL) had a good friend helping her get back in shape after her pregnancy. Because Mercedes could not afford a gym membership, her friend came over after work three times a week to go walking together. For women like Mercedes and Sarah, reliability and emotional connection—not specialized health knowledge—were what made peers desirable sources of support.

In other cases, low-income women forged close connections with peers who had similar-aged children. Like middle- and upper-class mothers, they bonded over shared experiences and appreciated having peers who could empathize with their struggles. Unlike middle-class mothers, none described these relationships in terms of shared parenting philosophies or health expertise. Becky Baker (white, twenty-six, LL) told me about how she hated breastfeeding—so much so that it made her question whether she was a good mother and whether she should have any more children. Her emotional anguish only abated when she was able to speak to her sister-in-law about her feelings: "She just had a baby too, so we were both really going through the same [thing]. She helped me deal with it a lot, and feel comfortable with the fact that this is the way it feels and it's not wrong to feel that way, because everyone feels that way." For Becky, support from a mother in a similar situation to her own became critical for helping her overcome feelings of despair and alienation from her body following the birth of her child. And Kathryn Schmidt (white, twenty-four, LL) felt so close to her friend Jen—also a single mom—that they were considering getting an apartment and raising their children together. Kathryn explained, "[Jen's] just very down to earth. She's got two kids. She just had her second baby, and she's just very down to earth and mature and responsible. Her and I, we haven't known each other that long. I just met her not even a year ago, but . . . if I couldn't go to my mom, she's the other person I would [ask about health]." As Kathryn admitted, they had known each other less than a year, but she explained, "You know in a relationship when you feel like you've known somebody forever? That's how it is with her. Like, I feel like I've known her forever, and I can definitely count on her." Kathryn and Jen had a relationship that was closer than what most other women described, almost like family; nevertheless, their relationship epitomizes what many poor and working-class women looked for in supportive relationships with their peers: solidarity, dependability, and the ability to bond over shared experiences.

## Conclusion

Sociologists studying motherhood in the contemporary United States have argued that now, more than at many points in the near and distant past, women are expected to do more for their children with less social support.[16] The continued idealization of the nuclear family form in popular culture and policy initiatives places a premium on family units comprised of married parents and their dependent children living together, even though the number of children living in such households has declined over the years.[17] New and recently revived childrearing trends like extended breastfeeding and attachment parenting insist that optimal child outcomes can only be achieved when at least one parent—usually a mother—is devoted to caring for children full-time. Furthermore, the declining birth rates, delayed childbearing, and medicalization of pregnancy and childbirth that predominate in many US communities mean that women often have little exposure to the events of maternal embodiment or to children prior to becoming mothers themselves. Thus, it is no surprise that so many US mothers feel surprised by the things that happen to their bodies during pregnancy, childbirth, and the postpartum period. It is also no surprise that these women often feel socially isolated and overwhelmed by the physiological and cultural demands of new motherhood in a society that holds them solely responsible for the health and development of their babies.

At the same time, social relationships remain critical to women's reproductive body projects. The relationships that women gravitate toward—and the forms these relationships take—are patterned by class. Middle- and upper-class women tended to approach these relationships instrumentally, building relationships with peers and healthcare providers who shared and supported mothers' health and body values. These women usually placed a premium on developing their own health knowledge and expertise—whether in addition to or as an extension of their professional identities—and they sought out horizontal social relationships in which they could access valuable advice while having their own expertise taken seriously. In contrast, poor and working-class mothers were more open to receiving health and body advice in vertical relationships with people they believed to have greater knowledge than themselves: WIC counselors, physicians, and their own mothers. They also emphasized personal connection and attention in determining whom they turned to for support—citing long-standing relationships with family or unusually attentive care from health professionals— rather than the consumerist approach to selecting relationships on the basis of having the "right" health values that middle- and upper-class women favored. Meanwhile, most poor and working-class mothers did not see their peers as optimal sources of health advice; some disregarded peers whom they viewed as having deficient values, while others cherished close friends for the emotional support they could provide (but not necessarily for their specialized body-care knowledge).

The experiences of mixed-class women shed further light on these patterns. Annie Castro, Gita Potter, and Nicki Lindsay were all mothers from middle-class backgrounds with college degrees who were eligible for WIC due to low income (HL). These women had made the decision to stay at home to raise their children, and their husbands—Annie's, a teacher, Gita's, a medical student, Nicki's, a pastor—were college educated but currently earning little money. As their comments in this chapter make clear, however, these women had a lot in common with HH women in terms of their cultural values and health practices. Gita described WIC's health guidelines as "simple," and Annie bemoaned the fact that WIC food vouchers did not apply to the organic products she had researched and decided were optimal for her family. Nicki recounted a story about attending a roundtable discussion at WIC where, even though she was a WIC client, she positioned herself as a breastfeeding advocate and an ally of the WIC staff member running the session. In this way, she sought to establish the kind of horizontal relationship with health providers that many middle-class women also described to me.

In contrast, Cass Blackwell and Louise Peralta were upwardly mobile mothers from working-class backgrounds; both were financially too well off to qualify for WIC or other assistance programs, but neither had a college degree. Cass and Louise both attempted to participate in "mommy groups," the social networks that many middle-class women described as central sources of peer-to-peer health information and support, but with mixed success. For Louise, attending an in-person meetup of a mothers' group she had participated in online brought painful reminders of the social exclusion she had faced as a working-class "country" kid growing up and going to school in "town"; in spite of the many experiences she shared with these women as mothers of similar-aged children, she still sensed an intangible social distance that was hard to bridge. Cass had more success joining a support group for mothers with postpartum depression, even forming a new friendship with one of the other women in the group: cosmopolitan, trust fund–supported Emily Fischer. The dynamic of their relationship, however, was more hierarchical than most of the friendships middle-class women described to me. Over the course of our joint interview, I witnessed Cass consistently defer to Emily's confidently expressed knowledge and expertise. In this way, Cass seemed willing to take on the position of knowledge recipient—rather than knowledge expert—in a somewhat vertical relationship, similar to how poor and working-class mothers in my study related to medical professionals or to older, more experienced mothers.

These findings from mixed-class mothers suggest that educational attainment and class background in childhood—both of which figure strongly into *cultural capital*—are stronger predictors of mothers' orientations toward health knowledge in social relationships than is current financial position. In other words, the socialization and cultural tastes that women held as a result of their class upbringing influenced both the type of health literacy they held and the social contexts in which they encountered health information. To be clear, higher levels of engagement with health-related discourses did not always yield more beneficial health practices; as described earlier, middle- and upper-class women's faith in their own ability to "do [their] own research," coupled with homogenous social groups that reinforced those convictions, sometimes led to unhealthful practices like vaccine refusal. Nevertheless, the ways in which highly educated mothers arrived at their decisions about health—by gathering information and consulting with friends and medical providers as equals—helped to secure their social position as moral, knowledgeable citizens committed to the ideology of healthism. Poor and working-class mothers who accessed health and body-care information through vertical relationships may have gotten helpful advice—indeed, there is something to be said for listening to the suggestions of people with greater experience or professional training than oneself!—but, in accepting a subordinate position vis-à-vis advice givers (health professionals or their own mothers), they may also have cemented their status as being less knowledgeable, less independent, and less expert.

Among poor and working-class mothers, a second pattern emerged according to race and ethnic background: white mothers in the low-income group were more likely to cite positive and supportive relationships with their peers, though they attributed the importance of these relationships more to their emotional closeness generally than to specific body-care values or knowledge they believed their friends to have. In contrast, Black and Latina low-income mothers overwhelmingly discounted their peers as helpful sources of support in making health and body-care decisions, preferring expert medical advice or help from their own mothers whenever possible. These racial/ethnic differences in utilization of peer support are based on fairly small numbers of respondents and should thus be treated as provisional, but they raise questions for further study.

Lastly, in my interviews with many low-income mothers of color, my questions about health and body-care goals were met with answers about women's financial and educational ambitions. As I will discuss in future chapters, this suggests that "health" may not occupy the same position in guiding all mothers' decisions about how to raise their children; instead, different cultural and material concerns may make "health" a greater or lesser priority in mothers' decision making.

2

# The Gender of Wellness

*The Labor of Body Care Falls to Mothers*

Fiona Garcia, a white, upper-middle-class mother in California, had recently given birth to her second child when I came to her home for an interview. Fiona was already in her midthirties when she met her husband, Carlos, and she told him, in no uncertain terms, what her priorities were: "I said, 'You've got a timeline. I'm going to be forty. I want at least two kids, so we've got to get going!'" Luckily, Carlos was on board. Although it took Fiona and Carlos more than a year after they married to conceive their first child, now, at age thirty-nine, Fiona had a twenty-two-month-old son and a seven-week-old daughter. Caring for two children under age two was daunting, though. Carlos's job did not offer much in the way of paternity leave, so Fiona's parents took turns coming to stay and help out. Fiona appreciated their help, but her account of each grandparent's visit revealed a stark gender divide in the way heterosexual couples manage caring work. "My dad was here, and he literally forgot to put a meal for me on the table while [my newborn daughter] was screaming. . . . I ended up making myself a [microwaveable] chicken dinner. Like, 'Dad, are you serious? You came here to help me and this is what you did?' He fed himself, and he had invited a friend over and they were having a great time, drinking wine, and talking away. Meanwhile, [my son is] screaming and he had to go to bed, and the baby's screaming. Nobody's like a mom." Fiona's father fully intended to help: it was the whole purpose of his visit. But he simply did not notice—or did not recognize as his responsibility—the fact that Fiona needed dinner or that one of his grandchildren was screaming and overtired. I asked Fiona what her mother did when she visited, and Fiona responded, "Everything. Anything that I would do, she would do. Laundry, picking up, putting the kids to bed, holding them, feeding them, playing with them. . . . My dad's great at making a dinner and feeding the dog, but he can't get either child to be entertained."

Fiona's description of her parents' different caregiving styles was about more than two grandparents with different strengths. In concluding that "nobody's like a mom," Fiona was highlighting a pattern of gender differences in recognizing and responding to others' needs: while her father could take responsibility for discrete tasks, her mother was better at noticing what needed to be done and then doing it without having to be asked. In essence, Fiona's mother acted as a near-seamless extension of Fiona herself, whereas her father became an additional responsibility she had to manage.

The *noticing* that Fiona describes her mother doing is one of three domains of gendered body-care disparities that this chapter will discuss, alongside *information gathering* and *supervising*. These responsibilities entail, respectively, paying attention to the bodily needs of others; assembling information about how best to care for children's health and bodies; and planning and overseeing any care that others provide. This wellness work is neither naturally nor exclusively the province of women. Nevertheless, in interview after interview, women in heterosexual couples reported that they had become the default providers of wellness-related family labor. This chapter asks how such arrangements develop.

As the previous chapter discussed, mothers look to their networks of family, friends, and professionals to learn how to care for their own bodies and their children's bodies during and after pregnancy, culminating in the development of *reproductive body projects*. Class affects whom they rely on most: poor and working-class mothers are more likely to turn to their own mothers; middle-class mothers often prefer to trade tips with "mom friends" of similar age, values, and demographics; and both groups draw on medical expertise, but in distinct ways. Throughout these women's accounts, though, one potential source of support was glaringly absent: their male partners.

That absence was not due to an absence of men in these women's lives. All thirty middle- and upper-class mothers I interviewed were married; eleven of fourteen mixed-class mothers were married. And of twenty-six poor and working-class women, about two-thirds were married (nine) or living with boyfriends (eight). White mothers were more likely to be partnered than women of color, and higher-class women were more likely to be partnered than those with lower incomes or levels of education. But while rates of marriage and cohabitation varied across groups, most women had husbands or boyfriends with whom they could, in theory, coparent and discuss their health concerns. In reality, when I asked mothers whom they turned to for advice and support in making health and body-care decisions, male partners rarely made the list.

Some of the reasons for this omission may be pragmatic. When women sought advice about health or childrearing questions, they often looked to people with more parenting experience than themselves; in most cases, their partners were equally new to raising children, and thus lacked the expertise that might make them helpful sources of advice. But when it came time for someone in the household to take the lead on gathering advice and other information—to become an expert—most couples defaulted to putting mothers in charge of family health.

The first section of this chapter will explore the various ways women took responsibility for noticing, gathering information, and supervising provision for children's body-care needs. These stories include discussions about how couples did (or did not) negotiate that responsibility, how they rationalized their division of labor, and their various frustrations with and/or resignation to their current situation. The second and third sections of the chapter will ask about how and when women are made responsible for this work. There, I argue that assigning women responsibility for family health needs does not begin in motherhood but, instead, has its roots in the body-conscious socialization that most women experience beginning in childhood. When women become mothers, parenting advice taps into this preexisting socialization, framing women as the most natural, inevitable bearers of health and body-care responsibilities. And while race and class may influence the size of this gender gap in body-care labor, the presence of the gap persists in households across race and class lines.

## Gender and Caregiving Responsibilities

### Noticing

One of the primary gender differences that mothers in my study described in how they and their male partners approached caregiving was in what I call *noticing*: observing that a child seems hungry or sleepy, or tracking changes in children's bodies and behavior that could herald a health problem or a new developmental stage. A brief personal example: when I gave birth in 2018, the hospital provided my spouse and me with a chart, directing us to spend those first, sleep-deprived days of our child's life carefully documenting the quantity and contents of every diaper we changed to make sure she was drinking enough milk. Admittedly, we are both habitual list makers, so this was a task we felt well suited to performing. By the time we brought our new baby home, we were primed to apply that kind of detail-oriented noticing to the various functions of her tiny body.

Some of the body-focused noticing that caregivers do is elective; the detailed logs of diaper changes that we dutifully kept may have provided doctors with helpful clues had our child become unwell, but since her early days were healthy and uneventful, these documents served little purpose beyond conditioning us to keep track of everything. A great deal of caregivers' noticing, however, is more unambiguously necessary: noticing whether a child's fussiness can be explained by hunger or teething or whether, perhaps, it is a sign of impending illness; noticing the antsy body language of a potty-training toddler about to have an accident.

Marjorie DeVault explains how this sort of noticing—which she calls "attention"—gets gendered, writing, "Attention does not come naturally to mothers; it develops from both loving concern and the very strong societal prescription that mothers are responsible for their children's well-being."[1] In the story that opened this chapter, both of Fiona's parents loved their grandchildren, but only one of them—Fiona's mother—had learned to express that love by noticing what needed doing and taking care of it unbidden. How did Fiona and other women make sense of such disparities?

Many women I spoke to took on the bulk of body-care-related work in their families following the birth of a child. Often, they explained these arrangements in terms of the physiological sex differences that rendered cisgender men unable to bear children or breastfeed. Fiona, whose husband's job meant that he was often away during and after her pregnancy, described how she had come to rely on a community of mothers to make sense of her pregnancy symptoms: "Being a mom is a common thing, right? People do it every day, all around the world. So it's a new experience for you, but there's a gazillion people you can ask about it. So it's always nice to be able to have somebody to talk to who's been through the same thing. My husband has no idea. He wouldn't notice. And even if he did—if you told him—he'd be like, 'Oh, okay.' [Laughs] Because that's not something he will ever experience."

Fiona believed her husband might be able to intellectually grasp information about the embodied elements of motherhood but, without having lived through those experiences in his own body, he would never be able to fully understand or empathize with her. Similarly, Amy Chen (thirty-five, Asian, HH) recounted the stark gender division in caregiving labor and awareness that she faced with her husband, a professor: "[My husband] didn't take a paternity leave, so I did everything on my own, basically, right from the start. My son was born on September 3, and guess what? Class started that week, so there was no way that he could not teach class. I thought he could pass it on to a TA, but it didn't happen. So I was basically on my own when it came to that."

Although Amy assured me that she appreciated "all the work and all the support I get from my husband," she added, "Having girlfriends that *really* know what you're going through . . . that you can talk to and share things with, I think that really helps." Both Amy and Fiona believed that fathers' empathy and support—while welcome—were no substitute for having lived through the embodied experiences of pregnancy, childbirth, and breastfeeding, at least when it came to understanding mothers' physical concerns.

Yet even if most husbands and boyfriends could not empathize with these bodily experiences and sensations, they might, nevertheless, still be involved as full coparents by providing mothers with emotional support and, once children were born, doing their share of feeding, washing, and decision making. For most women I interviewed, that level of equality never arrived, and most mothers remained primarily responsible for issues related to children's health and bodies.

Shontel Sykes (Black, twenty, LL) lived with her boyfriend and two children, a three-year-old and a newborn. She told me, "I would love for somebody to just make me a meal, because I'm always making food for everyone. I cook for everyone in my family, so I would like for somebody else to cook and for me to sit back and rest and enjoy it and not have to worry about it." I asked about her boyfriend's contributions, and she noted that while he was able to make breakfast, that was about as far as his homemaking skills extended. She added, "He's not a neat freak like I am. He's more of 'I'll put it back wherever I want to put it back.' And I'm like, 'It doesn't go there, it goes here.' We argue about it!" Being a "neat freak," as Shontel put it, meant *noticing* the usual places where household objects were stored and keeping those consistent, to better help other members of the household find things. Shontel's boyfriend's inability or unwillingness to do that kind of noticing became a source of conflict within their relationship, and it meant that Shontel ended up doing the bulk of the housework. Similar to the families that Arlie Hochschild and Anne Machung describe as crafting "family myths" about housework, couples like Shontel and her boyfriend often embrace narratives that explain their unequal workload in terms of women's pickiness or greater propensity to notice dirt and disorder, rather than in terms of men's passive resistance to doing their share of childcare or housework.[2]

In short, the gender division in noticing translates into a gender division in caregiving and household labor: the person who notices a task that needs doing becomes the person responsible for seeing that it gets done. Women, who are socialized to notice others' needs—even to anticipate them—are thus more likely to do the work that follows from noticing (or to have to ask someone else to do it, which becomes work, too). Some men, meanwhile, may cite maternal instincts to explain why their female partners attend more closely to children's needs, or they may fall back on myths about male "dirt blindness" that relieve them of responsibility for noticing housework that needs to be done.[3] Indeed, some women—like Shontel, Amy, and Fiona—may even reinforce those views as they rationalize men's inability to understand.

### Information Gathering

A second, related area where gender divisions showed up was *information gathering*. As many mothers recounted, parenthood brings an endless string of choices to make, and "good parents" approach those choices by "doing their research": middle- and upper-class mothers, especially, described taking classes, reading books, or finding a favorite parenting podcast or blog that aligned with their preferred parenting philosophy. Among poor and working-class parents enrolled in WIC, it was primarily mothers, not fathers, who attended the program's health and nutrition classes. And while the *quality* of the information women gathered was mixed—especially among those who sourced advice from peers and random websites—many (especially HH) women emphasized the importance of *quantity*, asserting that more information would help them make better, more informed choices.

Grace Potter (white, twenty, LL) lived with her parents, four sisters, and toddler nephew, as well as her fiancé and their infant son. She told me that she and her mother did most of the cooking for the household; they were able to afford fresh produce and other healthful foods because Grace and her sister Whitney—both mothers of young children— received WIC benefits along with a supplemental farmer's market credit. Grace described WIC's influence on her household: "I think they [WIC] know that if we have twenty bucks we're going to go out and buy pizza. So they're like, 'Well here's a healthy alternative.' I think that's what WIC does: it gives you a healthier alternative, and it's something that you can stick to, and you can change your lifestyle." Grace spoke approvingly of the scientifically supported literature that WIC provided, adding, "[WIC] gives you stuff to back it up. It's not just hearsay, they back it up." In this way, she signaled her preference for evidence-based advice when it came to health and body-care practices. Grace recounted, also, her own enthusiastic research into healthy foods for her baby: "I get the parent magazines, the baby magazines, and there's articles in there on healthy snacks for my son. I mean, he can't eat them yet, but I save them. . . . And I'd rather make real bananas and stuff that I can mash up, now, than the baby food, because they put stuff in it to keep it from spoiling."

Feeding work—and the invisible labor of learning about nutrition, evaluating evidence, and selecting groceries that it entailed—seemed to fall mainly on the women of the household, Grace included. While she never mentioned her fiancé's role in this work, their negotiation over a separate issue—where to baptize their son—indicated how the couple drew on gendered roles and expectations to make decisions about their child. Grace explained, "He says because I'm the mom, in the long run, it makes more sense [for our son to go to church with me]. [My fiancé's] dad went to church with them up until they were like four and five. After they got their first communions, he didn't go to church with them.

So what would the point be in putting [my son] in a church where he wouldn't be going with his dad, and I don't speak enough Spanish to understand what's going on?" Although Grace's fiancé would have preferred to raise their son in his own, Spanish-speaking church, he ceded that decision to her because he saw her as primarily responsible for day-to-day caregiving and religious instruction. In the same way, many fathers ceded everyday health and nutrition decisions to mothers.

Charlotte Moran (biracial, thirty-two, HH) described introducing a bottle to her daughter, Lily; she offered this as an example of how she and her husband made health- and development-related decisions: "I'll usually have gotten a pretty good sense of what that's going to be like, based on books I've read, talking to friends, sometimes talking to Lily's teachers—she goes to daycare. And then I'll compile that information and talk to my husband about it." I asked Charlotte whether her husband supported her decisions, and she replied, "Yeah, because he hasn't done the research. He has no idea." Charlotte and her husband, both graduate students, believed in sharing domestic tasks—and both, certainly, had strong skills in gathering and evaluating evidence. But since Lily's birth, Charlotte had slipped into doing most of the cooking for the family and taking responsibility for investigating child-development and health questions as they arose.

Arrangements like those Charlotte and Grace described were fairly typical among my respondents, regardless of class or geographic location: mothers sought out (or received unsolicited) information about nutrition, medical care, exercise, and other issues pertaining to their own or their children's bodies. They then sorted through that information; assessed the health risks and benefits of one approach versus another; measured possible courses of action against their personal values, priorities, and budgets; and made a decision about how to proceed. In the case of "egalitarian" couples like Charlotte and her husband, women took on the additional labor of delivering the predigested data to their partners to maintain the narrative that they were making decisions together.

Lara Noble (white, forty, HH) explained why she and her husband tended to agree about parenting decisions: "Usually we're on the same page. . . . For the most part, Joe has always followed what I do, in large part because I'm the one that reads everything and probably cares more about it. I'm home more with them than he is." Her phrasing—"we're on the same page"—suggested that she and her husband shared childrearing decisions. But a closer reading ("he follows what I do because I'm the one that reads everything and probably cares more") tells a different story. Women like Lara, Charlotte, and Grace tended to do more noticing when it came to their children's health and development, often because they spent more time at home with their children. They were the primary interfaces with teachers and healthcare providers, and were more likely to be on the receiving end of parenting advice from friends and family members. These experiences sensitized them to upcoming developmental milestones and potential parenting challenges (giving a bottle to an exclusively breastfed baby, introducing solid foods, tackling potty training, and more), as well as exposing them to different approaches that they might take in meeting those challenges. And thus it fell to mothers to gather information: learning about different approaches, evaluating their merits, and distilling them for their male partner in a way that allowed both parents to maintain the fiction that they were equally involved in these choices.

## Supervising

The third dimension of women's disproportionate responsibility for health and body care is *supervising*. For many women, language describing husbands as "helping" or as reaching consensus often masked the fact that they had fallen into a fairly traditional, gendered division of labor: mothers took primary responsibility for children's care (both learning how to do it and ensuring that it got done), while fathers acted as their assistants. Unlike with pregnancy or breastfeeding, there was no biological reason why male partners could not do more of the work of daily body care or of researching developmental and health issues. Yet many couples continued to treat their responsibilities after children were born as a continuation of the division of labor that began during pregnancy: women were presumed to be more attuned to their children's bodily needs and well-being, with fathers taking on a supportive but unequal role.

Stephanie Brewer (white, thirty-two, HH) described a typical weekend morning with her husband. She attended a once-weekly yoga class on Sunday mornings and left her husband to feed the kids lunch. She had developed a system for introducing new foods to her children (a result of her information gathering), and she made her own baby food purées. She described the division of labor between herself and her husband thus: "I did all of the prep of making the food, ice cube traying it [into single-serving portions], sticking it in the freezer. I would say to my husband, 'Okay, feed Olive lunch, feed Danny lunch.' And my husband would be like, 'What haven't they eaten [yet this week]?'"

Even though Stephanie's husband was aware of the rotating food schedule she had devised—and even though he helped to maintain it when he was in charge of feeding the children—it was obvious that he viewed her as the final authority, while he acted as her deputy when she was away. Worth noting here is that Stephanie's feeding schedule was a variation of the "three-day wait rule," wherein some caregivers wait three to five days after introducing one new food before introducing another, in order to identify any food allergies their child might have. This approach, while supported by the American Academy of Allergy, Asthma, and Immunology for children who are at high risk for food allergies (especially when a parent or sibling has an allergy), is not routinely recommended for typically developing, healthy babies.[4] Nevertheless, this approach was popular among class-privileged women like Stephanie and her peers, a way to perform risk avoidance through work on their children's bodies. Husbands typically supported, but did not design, such feeding plans.

Viewing fathers as taking a supporting role was common across racial/ethnic and class lines. Juana Reyes (Latina, twenty-nine, HL), a doctoral student and mother of one, also described her husband as a helper. She explained, "My husband does help, but I think because I am the primary caregiver he hasn't had to be too firm with our son. He will say things like, 'Remember Mommy said not to do that.'" By citing Juana's authority, her husband reinforced—for both himself and their son—that Juana, not her husband, was the primary parent. And while women's supervisory role was something many couples tried to downplay (such as when mothers gathered all the information and then presented it to their husbands so they could be involved in decision making), at other times that role was readily apparent.

## Racialized Class and the Division of Body-Care Labor

The stories described above illustrate a pervasive gender gap in body-care work, where women—regardless of class—shoulder a disproportionate amount of responsibility for family wellness. But previous research suggests that racial and ethnic differences, in combination with class, may matter when it comes to the gendered division of housework. Do these differences carry over into body care?

Earlier studies that have asked heterosexual couples to record their daily contributions to housework found that, while women in all racial/ethnic groups do more housework than men, on average, the size of the gender gap varies across groups. Specifically, Black heterosexual married couples have the smallest gap in hours spent on "core" housework (i.e., chores like food preparation that must be done regularly and consistently, as opposed to sporadic tasks like yard work and vehicle maintenance). Some authors have pointed to the role of gender socialization for Black boys or the sons of low-income single mothers, which links competence at household chores (including those often stereotyped as feminine) to successful adult masculinity and might drive men to participate more fully in cooking and cleaning work alongside their partners.[5] Others conclude that the relatively small gender gap in housework time is due not to Black men's assuming more responsibility for core chores but to the fact that Black women, particularly those with higher earnings, spend *less* time on cooking and cleaning than do women of other racial/ethnic groups. As Liana Sayer and Leigh Fine write, "Black women's lower levels of housework at all levels of earnings vis-à-vis other women points to the reduced salience of housework as a means of doing gender in Black married couples."[6] In other words, in Black women's own self-conceptualization and priorities, responsibility for wellness and housework may be less central to their sense of femininity and good motherhood, sometimes taking a back seat to other priorities like economic provision.

There is some evidence for Sayer and Fine's conclusions in my study. I did not ask respondents to keep time diaries, nor did I interview their partners about the division of labor in their relationships. But several mothers' stories hinted at widely differing degrees of investment in nonessential body-care labor. Middle- and upper-class mothers, most of whom were white, tended to offer lengthy, highly detailed accounts of the health and body-care projects they undertook on behalf of their children. These women did much more housework and childcare than their husbands, but it is not clear whether all of their excess labor was *necessary* to ensuring children's healthy development.

By contrast, poor and working-class mothers, many of whom were Black and Latina, were more likely to give shorter, more matter-of-fact answers that explained their bodily practices and aspirations but did not linger over the details of how and why they made these choices. Instead, their answers frequently referenced the other things in their lives that took priority: work, caregiving, negotiating transportation logistics, and more. LaDonna Douglas (Black, eighteen, LL) was one such mother. A star basketball player whose father, older brother, and older sister had attended college on athletic scholarships, she found her own plans for upward mobility via athletic scholarship sidetracked when she got pregnant the previous year. Now, back on the team and working to get in top shape for her senior high school season, she noted the challenges of doing this while caring for an infant: "It's kind of hard with a kid, because I can only do some things when I have him." Still, when I asked her to reflect on how she felt about her health practices overall, or whether she might wish to do anything differently, she replied, "I feel good about it. . . . I think I'm doing a good job how I'm doing it now." LaDonna was similarly matter-of-fact when I asked her about other health-related topics like breastfeeding or dietary changes during pregnancy; while she recounted conversations with her doctor and family members about these choices, she did not seem particularly interested in developing them into a full-scale reproductive body project. Instead, she was most animated and passionate when she spoke about her ambitions: to have a competitive basketball season and get recruited to play in college. And when she spoke about her son's future, she added, "I want him to be athletic. I want him to do sports, be active." This was a matter of good health, but more importantly, in Douglas family tradition, a way of parlaying athleticism into socioeconomic opportunity.

It is possible that interactions like the one I had with LaDonna reflect class and cultural differences in conversational style or, perhaps, differences in rapport (because I was a white, middle-class researcher, perhaps interviewees with identities similar to mine felt more at ease to speak at length). And age certainly plays a role, too: many lower-income women I spoke to were also fairly young (in their teens and early twenties), just getting started in their working lives at the same time as becoming mothers. But I would suggest that, alongside these potential contributing factors, middle- and upper-class women *did* spend more time on health-related projects because they *had* more time for that work. Past research has found that higher-income people tend to engage in more leisure-time exercise, rely less on time-saving take-out and prepackaged meals to feed their families, and be better able to afford the food waste that comes with introducing unfamiliar or challenging foods to children.[7] Poor and working-class mothers, in contrast, must manage feeding their families in the face of additional, often unpredictable challenges: lack of access to nearby, high-quality grocery stores, unreliable appliances or electricity, intermittent work schedules, and more.[8] Several authors have noted that increases in wives' and mothers' leisure time are often accompanied by cultural demands that they reinvest that time into their children and households.[9] Indeed, far from being medically necessary or even ideal, many HH women's reproductive body projects (such as Stephanie Brewer's meticulous approach to introducing new foods) served primarily to demonstrate their care for their children and their ability to adopt complex or time-consuming routines: all markers of social status. These findings suggest that white, middle- and upper-class mothers spend more time on body projects than their working-class peers. And as a result, it seems likely that the gender gap in body-care labor may be wider in white, middle-class households than in the households of many of the poor and working-class families I studied. The question we turn to next asks, How do women learn to perform this work, and when does that learning begin?

## Developing Feminine Body Consciousness

### "I knew a lot about nutrition from my bulimia days": Pre-pregnancy Body Consciousness

For many women in my study, learning about nutrition, exercise, and other body-care practices predated their transition into motherhood. Nearly all respondents had stories to tell about a moment, often in adolescence, when they started to feel self-conscious about their appearance and learned to conceal or modify their bodies in response. Chevonne Lewis (Black, twenty-three, LL) recalled, "I was always scrawny, and I got picked on some for that. I started filling out in eighth grade, and I did cheerleading, but I was still always self-conscious. I've never been completely comfortable with showing myself, even in the gym locker room." Following the births of her sons, Chevonne said that she had stopped worrying about her appearance, but that she would like to start exercising more: "I'm not someone who cares about a certain number on the scale, but I'd like to make my body stronger and more flexible."

Like Chevonne, Diane Sperry (white, thirty-seven, HH) recalled getting teased for being skinny as a child. Her unfavorable body image continued into the present; she admitted that she tried to avoid looking in the mirror whenever she could. Yet Diane also resented society's focus on looks, particularly the amount of work it would take to make her body align with mainstream beauty norms: "As much as I dislike myself, I also don't like to spend a lot of time on appearance. It's not a priority to dress up in the perfect clothes and put on the perfect makeup and have my hair done perfectly. It's important to me not to spend time on those things." Whereas Diane and Chevonne faced teasing for being skinny, Lara Noble (white, forty, HH) traced her body image issues to chubbiness during adolescence and her mother's critiques, which, she felt, had caused her to develop an eating disorder. She explained, "I knew [my bulimia] was directly related to my mom. She had been this tall, thin person. I think it rocked her world to have a girl that was not. And she just made enough comments that I internalized that. But I hated the mental jail—that's what it felt like—of spending 90 percent of my waking hours thinking about food, weight, calories, exercise."

With the help of a therapist, Lara recovered from her eating disorder, but elements of that mindset remained with her into motherhood. She noted that she did not make many dietary changes when she became pregnant because "I'd been a healthy eater pretty much my whole life. I knew a lot about nutrition, mostly from my bulimia days." Although Lara seemed to recognize that bulimia was *not* healthy, she nevertheless equated the dietary habits she learned in her "bulimia days"— limiting calorie-dense foods, for example—with a healthy approach to pregnancy. And Lara was not alone in that attitude. Bree Turner (white, thirty-three, HH) described the lingering effects of anorexia from high school—a time, she said, when controlling her body became a way to manage her feelings of being insecure and out of control in her social life. She explained, "I thought high fat was bad, so I would eat bread and an apple for lunch and be starving. . . . I would be very focused on food, thinking about it all the time because I was hungry and bored. But then I would limit myself . . . so I never got that satisfaction." Like Lara, Bree spoke of her eating disorder both as something in the past and as an experience informing her present: "And then, I came out of it and learned a lot more about nutrition and metabolism. . . . I think it's never gone away. [My body has] always been something I've been aware of. I just know a lot more, now, about nutrition. I feel like I have more power, more control over it, because I can exercise." For Bree, moving past disordered eating seems to have meant swapping out one method of bodily self-control—restrictive eating—for another: exercise.

For many women, growing into adulthood meant reckoning with others' judgments and demands on their bodies, including the demand that they work on their bodies as projects in pursuit of beauty standards. They recognized—and resented—the amount of time and mental energy these projects required (which Lara called "mental jail"), and described trying to resist these demands in various ways. Yet the self-consciousness they had developed, the habit of viewing their bodies as objects that were somehow separate from their selves, remained.

This bodily alienation is a major site of gendered oppression facing women, according to feminist scholars and cultural critics. At a time when women in the United States and around the world are seeing increased opportunities in the realms of politics, careers, and education, mainstream beauty norms demand that they spend large amounts of time perfecting their bodies. Yet, writes Susan Bordo, "Each hour, each minute spent in anxious pursuit of that [beauty] ideal . . . is in fact time and energy taken from inner development and social achievement."[10] The women I interviewed described this body consciousness as painful and distracting. Many recounted watching their own mothers go on restrictive diets—some, like Michelle Carter (white, twenty-nine, HH), even accompanied their mothers to Weight Watchers meetings when they were children. And several explicitly told me they wanted to protect their own daughters from going through what they had.

## *"I don't want what happened to me to happen to them": Gender and Bodily Vulnerability*

Not all women I interviewed spoke of their bodies with such unhappiness, but virtually all recalled feeling dissatisfied with their bodies at various points in their lives. This shared experience is unsurprising, given that contemporary US gender norms reinforce a heightened body consciousness among women. That consciousness includes awareness of how one's body looks, but it also extends to women's sense of bodily vulnerability.

Mixed-class Florida mother Louise Peralta (white, thirty-six, LH) addressed this vulnerability when she told me the story of her rape more than twenty years earlier. When Louise was thirteen, her older brother and some of his friends got her drunk on wine coolers. Louise lost consciousness, and when she woke up, one of her brother's friends was raping her. She recalled, "I knew what was going on and I tried to fight him, and he beat me up. He leaves. His buddy comes in, does the same thing. He leaves. His buddy comes in, does the same thing. And my brother's in the other room, right in the living room!" Later, Louise confronted her brother, demanding that he hold his friends accountable for the rape, but he responded by telling her that if she told anyone what happened, he would tell them she was asking for it. This trauma echoed across the years and shaped both Louise's relationship to her own body and her approach to parenting two daughters. As a mother, she said, she knew what could happen to girls. "When they are on the playground, we're right there, like five feet away. We don't talk to other moms or anything. We're focused on them, because I don't want what happened to me to happen to them." With regard to her own body, Louise explained, "I don't want people to look at me. . . . Every time when I was skinny people bothered me, men bothered me. And now nobody even looks at me because I'm the fat girl. I feel safer, I guess, being like that." For Louise, gaining weight felt like a way to protect herself, to retake control of her body's safety after the assault. Suzanne Walsh (white, thirty-five, HH) shared a story similar to Louise's: "I felt sexualized from a very young age, and then I resisted it. I started messing with food. I wanted to be totally strong and lean and powerful. I got that way. I was totally anorexic. And then as a way to deflect people's attention toward me, I was like 'I'll get them off my back.' So I started gaining weight, and then I became very bulimic."

Across classes and geographic locations, women like Louise and Suzanne—and numerous other women I interviewed—recounted trying to manipulate their bodies as a response to feelings of being out of control, particularly when being sexualized against their will. Gaining or losing weight became a tool for them to wrest back control: if, they reasoned, their bodies drew the wrong kind of attention, the only power they had was to change their bodies.[11]

Both Louise's and Suzanne's stories also hint at the bodily vulnerability that many women feel. In the United States, where one in three women will experience sexual violence at some point in her life (according to the federal Department of Health and Human Services),[12] the threat of sexual assault influences how many—probably most—women view their bodies and move through the world: what we wear, when and how we enter public spaces, how freely we express desire, and more. That hyper-awareness of risk is not limited to survivors of sexual violence; its reach extends to all potential victims—that is, virtually all women. Of course, women are not the only people who experience sexual violence. But for most women, sexualization and potential victimization are treated as an inevitability in a way that they typically are not for most men.

Gendered socialization also teaches women to view their bodies as fragile and at-risk in numerous smaller, everyday ways. Iris Marion Young refers to women's relationship to their bodies as "feminine body comportment," in which the body is experienced as subject (actor) and object (acted upon) simultaneously.[13] When women and girls play sports, for example, societal norms as well as gender-specific rules of the sport itself remind athletes that they must worry about getting hurt, which can impede the athlete's ability to focus on the activity at hand.[14] In preschools, teachers devote more time to managing girls' bodies (adjusting messy clothing or hair, urging them to sit still or quiet down, cautioning them away from getting hurt, etc.) than they do boys', allowing boys to maintain a looser, more relaxed attitude toward their bodies that carries over into adulthood.[15] And such attention can be racialized as well as gendered: Black boys' and girls' horseplay is more likely to be viewed by teachers as aggressive and/or sexual, becoming a target for disciplinary intervention.[16] "Consequently," writes Young, a woman "often lives her body as a burden, which must be dragged and prodded along and at the same time protected."[17] Whether one is worrying about how one's body looks or about what harm might be done to it, these gendered and racialized social norms teach women, from an early age, to maintain a preoccupation with the body and its management.

## Doing Health and Gender

In the opening chapter of this book, I introduced the term "healthism," which refers to an ideology that frames health not only as "a desired state, but . . . also a prescribed state and an ideological position."[18] Healthism holds everyone accountable for making choices that are geared toward preserving and enhancing the body's health—through, for example, the cultivation of reproductive body projects—and it allows us to pass moral judgment on those who act in ways that increase their risks of ill health. But while people spanning diverse identities and backgrounds face healthist norms, the consequences of this ideology differ according to gender and other identity characteristics.

As described above, women are encouraged to view their bodies as fragile and at-risk, and to engage in self-protective strategies as a result. In contrast, boys and men in the United States learn from an early age that they must meet risk bravely, even seek it out in order to avoid charges of "weakness, homosexuality, or femininity."[19] Men who appear overly focused on the body—whether in relation to its appearance, its health, or its safety—risk having their masculinity questioned, and so must downplay the time and attention they devote to the body's care. Wellness, body consciousness, paying attention to worrying symptoms, and seeking medical care—essentially, being aware of and limiting bodily risk—are framed as feminine concerns.[20]

Scholars term this phenomenon "doing health": the health-focused dimension of gender performance (or, "doing gender") that all people engage in that makes them legible as masculine or feminine members of society.[21] Clare Williams, for example, finds that children living with chronic illnesses like asthma and diabetes adopt gendered patterns of compliance with preventive measures like taking insulin or using an inhaler. While girls were more likely to adapt their behaviors and identities to best manage their illnesses, for many boys, "control over their personal and social identities as 'normal, healthy males' was more important than controlling potential episodic occurrences of asthma," and diabetic boys concealed their insulin use so that they could "pass" as nondiabetic.[22] Since physical strength and virility are tied to hegemonic notions of masculinity, many boys and men thus neglect or downplay health issues in hopes of retaining a desired social identity.

Of course, not everyone conforms to hegemonic notions of gender or the health and body-related practices that accompany them: some women will inevitably appear insufficiently attentive to health, some men will appear too concerned about health risks and wellness, and some people will challenge these binaries through their very gender identification. However, Candace West and Don Zimmerman, who originated the concept of "doing gender," offer an important clarification about what the "doing" of gender (or health) might entail: "To 'do' gender is not always to live up to normative conceptions of femininity or masculinity; it is to engage in behavior *at the risk of gender assessment*."[23] In other words, "doing gender" is less about the intentionality or success of an individual's gender performance than it is about social context: performing these actions in a setting where people will judge as them as successful or failed, normative or subversive. Similarly, I would argue that "doing health" does not entail that we will always live up to normative conceptions of how we should pursue good health or avoid risks to ourselves or our children; it means that we constantly act in the face of *health assessment*: regardless of our intent, we are held accountable to dominant healthist notions of appropriate behavior. Doing health is unavoidable in a society like the United States, where healthist ideology reigns. And when we do health, we may be judged as succeeding or failing in that work, regardless of how much meaning we personally assign to that project. Such judgments carry moral and potentially stratifying consequences, which will be discussed further in the next chapter.

## Gendering Responsibility for Others' Bodies

Social norms for pregnant embodiment build on and intensify gendered expectations for doing health: pregnant people are often said to be in a "delicate condition" and urged to avoid excessive physical or emotional strain, and prenatal care guidelines from authorities like the American

College of Obstetricians and Gynecologists call for regular monitoring of pregnant bodies through frequent doctor visits. These and other norms reinforce women's responsibility for bodily awareness. Some people frame pregnancy as a new way of experiencing the body, requiring new habits of self-care and risk consciousness. I argue, however, that what is required is an extension of the feminine body consciousness that most women learn long before they become pregnant. Wellness was already women's work; pregnancy and new motherhood build on and refine those skills.

### Worrying for Two: Expanding Women's Risk Consciousness to Their Children

Mixed-class Christine Webber (white, thirty-seven, HL) was living in Florida with her husband, four-year-old son, and eleven-week-old twins when I interviewed her. Christine developed gestational diabetes in each of her two pregnancies, and her oldest son had since been diagnosed with Type 1 diabetes. Managing these successive health challenges had fallen to Christine, who was also the family's sole breadwinner. Christine explained, "I was very intimidated by knowing that I was going to have to do this diabetic diet thing. . . . [My son] has to deal with it—he was diagnosed when he was two years old, so really his mom had to deal with it, watch every single thing he ate, counting his carbs, figuring out how much insulin to give. It just seemed like a mathematical nightmare to me." Once she worked with a diabetic counselor, who helped her simplify the process by focusing on carbohydrate servings, Christine realized that she already knew how to do this: "That made it a lot easier. I was familiar with looking at carbs because of the Atkins Diet which I had done a couple of years before. And I was familiar with looking at labels because of the Weight Watchers diet and counting points. So that was not a problem." Christine's husband, a graduate student, was nominally the primary caregiver for their children while Christine worked. But because of gendered expectations—and, perhaps, Christine's prior experience with dieting—the management of their son's specialized diet fell to her.

Christine was not unique among my respondents. At the same time as women develop self-consciousness and risk-averse attitudes for their own bodies, cultural norms teach them to notice and care for the bodies of others as well. Susan Bordo theorizes that "women, besides *having* bodies, are also *associated* with the body, which has always been considered woman's 'sphere' in family life."[24] Simone de Beauvoir famously lamented this situation as "immanence," wherein women, in their roles as mothers and housewives, spend every day attending to the physical needs of others and have no energy left for creative, "transcendent" projects and careers.[25] And in her empirical study of feeding as "women's work," Marjorie DeVault found that household meal preparation and other duties associated with the direct care and nourishment of the body were associated with women and femininity, even in families where women work full-time and other kinds of housework are increasingly shared. These tasks require women to practice *attentiveness* (or "noticing"): not just performing finite chores around the home but expending constant mental energy to keep track of family members' bodily tastes, appetites, and needs. DeVault explains, "The physiological experience of pregnancy—and all of the explicit teaching that surrounds it—enforces attention to feeding: a woman learns that she provides, very directly, the nourishment that carries the fetus to term. Attention to children's sustenance continues as they grow. Even when the physiological connection of pregnancy has ended, mothers are still usually more responsible than fathers for feeding their children. They watch them develop, and consider their responses to food."[26] The notion that such attention to the bodies of others is learned is supported by both scholarly and popular writing. The bestselling pregnancy book *What to Expect When You're Expecting* introduces its take on the ideal pregnancy diet by offering the following advice: "You've got nine months' worth of meals and snacks . . . ahead of you—each one of them an opportunity to feed your baby well before he or she is even born. So open wide, but think first. . . . Remember that each bite during the day is an opportunity to feed that growing baby of yours healthy nutrients."[27] In this passage, the authors exhort pregnant people to extend their body consciousness to their future offspring by scrutinizing "each bite during the day." It does not seem like a stretch to point out that this hyperconscious approach to eating echoes the calorie-counting mindset many women develop as they grow into adulthood, often as part of eating-disordered thinking. As Bree Turner, whose adolescent eating disorder was described in the previous section, put it, "I think [my anorexic mentality]'s never gone away. It's always been something I've been aware of. I just know a lot more, now, about nutrition. . . . [When I got pregnant] I really wanted to make sure I had the vitamins, the protein. I wanted to make sure I was doing everything I was supposed to do as a mom to make sure she had the best nutrients." Bree claimed to have moved past her troubled relationship to food, but, like Lara Noble, she believed that her experience with learning to control her body—first through a restrictive diet, then later through exercise—prepared her to have a healthy pregnancy. In other words, both professional advice givers and mothers themselves frame reproductive body projects as an extension of the dietary and exercise regimens that, as appropriately feminine women, they ought already to have learned.

As in *What to Expect*, other healthcare advice urges pregnant women to scrutinize their body-care choices on behalf of their fetus. In recent years, the view of maternal bodies as conduits for harmful substances has begun to encompass not only obvious risks like recreational drugs and alcohol but also everyday exposures to toxic chemicals like pesticides. Avoiding these exposures (say, by buying organic groceries) has become one more burden that women disproportionately bear; writes Norah MacKendrick, such "precautionary consumption" has become a requirement of good motherhood both during and after pregnancy.[28] Today, Deborah Lupton adds, "Risk is a central discourse among those that surround the pregnant woman."[29] This anxiety about women as vectors of risk to their unborn children now extends backward into the pre-pregnancy period, a phenomenon Miranda Waggoner terms "anticipatory motherhood": the view that women should manage their pre-pregnancy bodies in anticipation of eventually becoming pregnant. Waggoner notes that this discourse is often racialized: white-appearing and light-skinned women get represented as responsibly planning for pregnancy, while darker-skinned Black and Latina women are presented as at risk of unplanned—and, by implication, unhealthy—pregnancy. Yet regardless of demographic, public health messaging "positions all women of childbearing age as pre-pregnancy and exhorts them to minimize health risks to future pregnancies, even when conception is not on the horizon."[30]

Such was the case for Britta Larson (white, thirty-five, HH), who explained that she had few changes to make in her routines once she became pregnant because "I was kind of in pregnancy mode already. You know, preparing for it for years." For Britta, that meant cutting from her diet "anything white except potatoes" and trying to lose weight in hopes of improving her ability to conceive. In theory, the goal of "anticipatory motherhood" is to nurture beneficial health behaviors in the early first trimester, when many people do not yet realize they are pregnant; in practice, this approach adds yet one more layer of health and body consciousness even to nonpregnant women who are already keenly aware of their bodies as objects to be looked at and protected from risk.

In short, the lines between maternal embodiment practices and pre-pregnancy health and body care have been blurred in two directions. Today more than ever before, pregnancy and maternal health standards are being imposed onto nonmothers, applying heightened risk scrutiny to any woman of childbearing age: extending pregnancy-specific practices *backward* into the pre-pregnancy years (and including those who may never become pregnant). Simultaneously, popular pregnancy advice implicitly encourages pregnant women and mothers to draw on the bodily attitudes and habits they may have cultivated pre-pregnancy—including, sometimes, eating-disordered practices of calorie counting and assigning moral value to "good" and "bad" foods. Many women then bring these practices *forward* as they make the transition to motherhood, where they frame such habits as "healthy" when done for the sake of a child's well-being.

*"I've got to make sure he has enough brain power to be smarter than other kids": From Preventing Harm to Optimizing Health*

For the majority of women I interviewed, pregnancy did, indeed, mark a period of intensified awareness of their bodies and bodily risks. Jessie Wozniak (white, thirty-one, HH) ran through a list of some of the basic changes she made as she and her husband began to try for a baby: "I had been on prenatal [vitamins] from the first inkling that we might be thinking about getting pregnant. . . . Don't drink—kids tend to come out looking funny when you do. No smoking. Which I hadn't been doing. Keep your body healthy so you keep the baby healthy." Jessie had wanted children for as long as she could remember, but her husband, Cory, did not. Their twenty-month-old son was the result of what Jessie called "a weak moment. . . . I took advantage of it. Not, you know, got him drunk, but where he was like, 'Yeah, why not? Let's try it.'" Jessie had already begun taking prenatal vitamins when Cory agreed to try. She concluded, "Thank God we got pregnant right away, because he probably would have changed his mind!"

Many people, of course, become pregnant by accident and do not make these kinds of preparations. But among those like Jessie who are actively trying to conceive, weeding out any behaviors that might inhibit conception or harm an embryo is a common practice. Specifically, in her wry comment about babies who "tend to come out looking funny," Jessie was drawing on discourses of fetal risk that arose during the latter half of the twentieth century. In the early 1960s, the highly publicized fetal anomalies caused by thalidomide (a drug prescribed to alleviate morning sickness during pregnancy) led to greater scrutiny of the drugs prescribed to pregnant people. The 1980s brought heightened attention to the potentially fetus-endangering practices of US mothers themselves, with racialized moral panics over drug-addicted newborn "crack babies" and the introduction of alcoholic beverage labels in 1988 to warn pregnant people of the dangers of fetal alcohol syndrome.[31] And in the 1970s and '80s, stricter regulations on lead in paint and gasoline in the United States publicized the health risks of lead to children while successfully decreasing children's exposure.[32] Together, these and other campaigns to protect children and fetuses have sensitized US culture at large—and mothers in particular—to the environmental health risks children face before and after birth.

But Jessie, like many other women I interviewed, did not stop at avoiding these well-established risks. She also read up on practices that could help optimize her child's development, explaining, "When I was pregnant, there was a lot of new research out about omega-3s and DHA. . . . I was like, 'Oh my God, I've got to make sure he has enough brain power to be smarter than other kids.' And breastfeeding was part of that. [The research said] it's still the best way to make sure that he's getting all of those things that he needs for proper brain development."

As Jessie's story makes clear, many mothers' very real concerns about fetal *risks* are, today, increasingly wrapped up with concerns about maximizing development and conferring bodily *advantages* to children. This view, echoed and amplified in the popular press, is articulated in a 2010

*Time* cover story on the "fetal origins" of human health and behavior, entitled "How the First Nine Months Shape the Rest of Your Life."[33] Author Annie Murphy Paul reviews a growing body of research into the potential impact of prenatal environment on a child's subsequent health and life chances. That environment, according to Paul, is shaped not only by the nutrition, drugs, pollutants, and infections that enter the pregnant body but also by the "mother's health, stress level and state of mind."[34] Paul recognizes that these new findings might create stress for pregnant people, but argues for viewing them as an opportunity: "We're used to hearing about all the things that can go wrong during pregnancy, but as these researchers are finding out, *it's frequently the intrauterine environment that makes things go right in later life*" (emphasis added). In short, this is an increasingly biomedicalized perspective that (1) treats the fetus as an independent patient (while rendering the gestational parent an "environment") and (2) views the prenatal period as a time not only for risk prevention but also for health and lifestyle optimization.

Occasionally, respondents—always class-privileged women, usually white—spoke to me with enthusiasm about having the opportunity to invest in their child's growth during and after pregnancy. Such was the case for Greta Davies (white, forty, HH), who struggled with infertility before finally getting pregnant: "It becomes a project, especially when you really want the baby. You just are so happy. . . . You just completely cater to your body, it's just wonderful. I'd make dinner and I'd be in bed at eight o'clock, horizontal, reading, and then I'd be asleep by nine. I'd do my yoga, which is wonderful. You have decaf, you don't smoke or drink. . . . But it becomes a project, especially the older you get. Women who are older read everything, probably read too much. And you just cater to every little detail because you can."

Greta acknowledged that her reproductive body project was intense, noting that older first-time mothers like herself "probably read too much" about health and prenatal development. And, as will be discussed more in chapter 5, Greta's comment that "you cater to every little detail because you can" signals a highly classed belief in her own agency and control over her body. On the whole, Greta's repeated assertions that caring for her pregnant body was "wonderful" suggest that she viewed this work with excitement about future possibility, rather than with fear about the risks her child might face.

Most women I spoke to were less likely to describe reproductive body projects as "wonderful" than to describe this work with a mixture of anxiety (about risk) and obligation. Mixed-class Annie Castro (white, twenty-nine, HL) explained that "I've got nine months to be in the best health of my life to give my babies the perfect climate to grow in as possible. And if I can control something, I will." I asked Annie what sort of things she was trying to control, and she responded, "I did the prenatal vitamins, even before my pregnancy. I tried to get as many toxins out of our home [as I could], from cleaners to laundry detergent, even what I put on my skin. I won't dye my hair. I won't smoke. I won't drink. I won't eat the soft cheeses. I mean, if there's an ounce of [a substance] they're not really sure about, I just don't even do it. I can give up anything for my children and gladly do it."

Annie's account echoes both Greta's and Jessie's recitations of health risks to avoid and health opportunities to pursue during pregnancy, but she also makes explicit a theme that is implicit in many mothers' remarks: avoiding risk—even uncertain, unproven risk—has become a requirement of good motherhood. That requirement begins before pregnancy (what Waggoner terms "anticipatory motherhood") and ties the protection of children to an ethos of maternal self-sacrifice. As Annie put it, "I can give up anything for my children and gladly do it."

### "Women are the power broker in the house": Responsibilizing Working-Class Mothers at WIC

The social norms that led middle- and upper-class women to take on the lion's share of wellness work in their marriages were also apparent in my ethnographic fieldwork at offices of the Women, Infants, and Children (WIC) program for low-income families.[35] Joy, a nutritionist and lactation consultant in California, explained that in her work with mostly young, low-income women, she enjoyed reminding them that their caregiving work offered a sort of *power*: "Women are the power broker in the house, because the woman is the one that buys all the food. If I don't like to eat chicken, I will not buy chicken. So everybody else in the house will have to cope and eat whatever it is that I buy. . . . If you buy [healthy food] and cook it, even when you don't want to eat it, your family is exposed to that." Joy added, "If you have to get anything done in the family, come visit the woman, because she'll get it done." Joy's point—that being the one responsible for a task gives one more power to control how it gets done—is true. But it is also true that noticing family members' health needs, gathering information, and supervising other caregivers is just a lot of work. And women across classes are doing much more of that than their male partners.

Oddly, the gender dynamics of caregiving that position women as primary supervisors of family health and men as "helpers" show up even when the parent receiving WIC's nutrition education is a single father with custody of his children. Joy described her interactions with fathers in glowing terms: "Men are wonderful because . . . it's not their normal, natural role to nurture and take care of children. But believe me, they do a much better job because if you tell them what to do, they do it. . . . The man will always look at it as, 'This is not my role so I might as well listen.'" Florida WIC nutritionist Tracie voiced similar sentiments, explaining,

> I always praise when the dad comes in. I always say "Oh! It's good to see the whole family here." Sometimes the dad takes the backseat, when the mom's more involved, when I see both parents in the counseling session. But if it's primarily the dad, I notice that they are more hesitant, when you're counseling. I think they're more honest, too. They kind of tell you the truth, and they're not really sure what the "right thing" to say is, so they just tell you truth. Sometimes, with moms, they've come here and they know how the WIC appointments work, and they say, "Oh, my child doesn't drink juice, and we're doing everything right."

Both Joy and Tracie spoke approvingly of the fathers they counseled who were primary caregivers, often favoring them over the mothers and grandmothers they more commonly instructed. In the view they both shared, mothers tend to be more knowledgeable about health, which can make them stubborn (or even untruthful) when interacting with health authorities like WIC staff; fathers, in contrast, they viewed as relatively clueless (and, thus, more receptive to WIC advice). Ironically, even as Joy urged mothers to embrace their "power" as caregivers, she celebrated fathers who did what they were told; essentially, Joy, Tracie, and other nutritionists at WIC (almost entirely women) replaced wives and mothers as the female decision makers for these men, further solidifying men's status as "helpers."

Joy and other counselors' attitudes toward women who *did* claim primary authority over their children's health and bodies reveal a contradiction within WIC's mission: on one hand, women—not men—are treated as the default caregivers and decision makers in the realm of family wellness. On the other hand, those women are still expected to be deferential to government and health authorities, especially (but not only) when they are dependent on the government for financial support. That expectation of deference is common in social-welfare programs that disproportionately deal with low-income families. As Jennifer Reich finds while examining the interactions between social workers and families in the child welfare system, "Parents who do not act with deference, who do not communicate recognition of their own failings, who do not communicate a desire to improve, or who do not agree to the terms required for assistance are perceived to be either in denial or beyond rehabilitation."[36]

Older or more experienced mothers in WIC, who tended to feel more confident about their decisions, found these conflicting demands that they take responsibility and show deference to be deeply frustrating. The message these demands sent was that parents should be empowered to make decisions for their families' health, but empowerment was a gift that could only be bestowed by WIC or other health authorities.

The extent to which women had to confront—or could avoid—this sort of second guessing from health and medical authorities was a function of class (and, likely, race as well—something the next chapter will explore further). But while their specific contexts often differed, mothers across classes received variations on the same message: wellness is women's work.

## Conclusion

Across class and racial lines, the mothers I interviewed described caregiving arrangements in their households where women held primary responsibility for noticing the bodily needs of children (and, to a lesser extent, other household members). Whether the need was immediate (a diaper in need of changing; a cranky toddler overdue for a nap) or longer term (a potential allergy needing to be monitored; a nutritional deficit needing to be remedied), women tended to do the mental work of paying attention and noticing what needed to be done.

Noticing is closely tied to the other elements of wellness work: information gathering and supervising. After recognizing that a need exists, someone—typically a woman—must take responsibility for learning how to address that need and ensuring that it gets taken care of. This set of responsibilities involves mental and emotional labor beyond simply performing caregiving tasks (preparing a meal, changing a diaper). It requires vigilance, attentiveness, mental list making, and managing relationships with advice givers and, in many cases, family members and partners who must be delegated to carry out these tasks when the primary caregiver is not around.

Women's enthusiasm for this work varied considerably. While some, like Greta Davies, were excited to dive into the reproductive body projects and caregiving labor that came with a long-desired pregnancy, others were more ambivalent. Nadia Bernard (white, thirty-six, HH) explained to me the anxiety she experienced when she became unexpectedly pregnant with her first child: "I worried that my husband would be at work a lot. I just was worried that I wouldn't have enough support. And basically, it's true. I really don't." For Nadia, an immigrant who felt isolated and ill suited to motherhood, the bodily demands of being a primary caregiver were taking a toll. She held that responsibility not because she felt particularly eager or well qualified for it, but because she was physically present more with their child. This arrangement is common: women are more likely than men to have parental leave to stay home with a newborn, and—when couples decide that one parent should leave work to care for children on a more permanent basis—to be the parent whose career is put on hold.

Yet while gender divisions in caregiving labor and responsibility become pronounced once a baby is born, mothers' stories reveal that the origins of wellness work and reproductive body projects precede motherhood. When recalling childhood and adolescence, nearly every woman had a story to tell about how she learned to feel self-conscious about her body, to view her body as vulnerable, and/or to work on her body as a project. Even as a researcher who studies gender and body image in the United States (and who has personally experienced some of those same pressures as a girl growing up in this culture), I was shocked at how many respondents reported histories of eating disorders, or at least eating-disorder-adjacent feelings and behaviors. I was even more surprised that several women who explicitly identified as having had eating disorders went on to cite those histories as sources of diet and nutrition knowledge that they could use to *have healthy pregnancies.* The mental contortions required to reframe an eating disorder—a literal illness—as a resource for good health are breathtaking.

The fact that so many women do make this connection speaks to the existence of popular pregnancy and parenting advice that encourages them to draw on past practices as a way to prepare for motherhood. The same intense bodily scrutiny that causes so many women to learn to focus on their own weight, appearance, and other features becomes an asset for noticing changes or irregularities in the body of a child, particularly one who cannot yet verbalize their own needs. Learning to live with deprivation (as when on a restricted-calorie diet), to read nutrition labels on food, or to engage in exercise for the sake of "wellness"— all manifestations of healthism—are skills that can be translated into "good" pregnancy care, as expectant mothers learn to eliminate potentially harmful substances from their diets and adopt other "healthy" behaviors in order to promote the well-being of the fetus.

Women's attitudes toward the reproductive body projects demanded of them as mothers—and their ties to pre-pregnancy body consciousness—were decidedly mixed. Some experienced this expectation as empowering: whether through their biological role in nurturing a child's development during pregnancy, or through their social role as mothers afterward, they felt that they were uniquely qualified to ensure the well-being of their child and were proud of that work. For other women who did not find wellness work particularly enjoyable—or who lacked the time or financial resources to invest in elaborate body projects—the gendered expectation that they take on the household's body care was more taxing. For these women, that expectation came to feel like a source of inequality with male partners, or like a drain on their time that competed with other priorities like educational and career aspirations.

But while many of the stories in this chapter speak to the mundane, routine elements of wellness work—attending to and nurturing a child's growing body—wellness discourses often carry an undercurrent of fear: namely, the fear of health risks that could manifest in pregnancy or early childhood, and the vigilance mothers must exercise to protect their child from harm. As the next chapter will show, women's work at noticing, information gathering, and managing bodily risks becomes a major site of moral judgment and surveillance in the contemporary United States. And while virtually all mothers, regardless of race/ethnicity or class, experience gendered pressures to do wellness work, moral discourses about *risk* are ripe for creating hierarchies of mothers along class and racial lines.

# 3

## The Costs of Avoiding Risk

*Trust and Accountability*

Women face social pressure to oversee family health and wellness. Guided by popular advice manuals or by government agencies like WIC, women learn to translate pre-pregnancy body habits into practices that will benefit their children. But alongside the time and labor this work entails come emotional costs: worries about health risks, and worries about not measuring up to societal expectations for managing those risks. Suzanne Walsh (white, thirty-five, HH) described these feelings: "I watched out for fish [when I was pregnant]. I'm a vegetarian, but I eat a lot of seafood. So, I remember a few times I looked up on my iPhone and found out that I had just had mahi-mahi, which is the one fish you shouldn't have, because of the mercury. I even called the obstetrician, and she was like, 'That's fine.' But you worry about everything, and then there's this added pressure because the drama of the family is all playing out on the woman's body. So everything becomes these high stakes."

Noticing and gathering information about children's health needs is the foundation of women's wellness work, and risk awareness forms an especially fraught part of that project. Suzanne, a graduate student with a history of anorexia and bulimia, was already concerned about whether her body was healthy enough to support a pregnancy; her awareness that her choices could harm her future child as well made her feel deeply anxious. And so, even as her husband and doctor reassured her that she was doing a great job, she worried, "Am I going to fuck it up? Am I not eating enough? Am I eating too much?' It's all on the woman to do it right."

The process of bringing a new baby into being can be unpredictable, and all the money and hard work in the world cannot guarantee the outcome one hopes for. Whether attempting to conceive, ensuring a successful pregnancy, or raising a healthily developing child, many prospective parents—class-privileged women in particular—struggle with the realization that this process is not fully under their control. For Suzanne, as for many other women, the sense that she was both singularly responsible for the safety of her baby-to-be *and* that she did not have full control over the outcomes led to a constant state of low-level worry.

For those with the ability to pay, a range of diagnostic services and products aim to provide peace of mind: during pregnancy, diagnostic ultrasound and genetic testing seek to identify potential issues in fetal development; after babies are born, pricy monitoring gadgets like the SNOO (a fourteen-hundred-dollar bassinet that bills itself as "the safest baby bed ever made") and Owlet Smart Sock (which monitors an infant's oxygen level and heart rate while sleeping) claim to help parents prevent the risk of Sudden Infant Death Syndrome (SIDS). Products and services such as these capitalize on new parents' anxieties around risk: anxieties that their child might come to harm, and anxieties that they are not doing all they could to prevent it.

This chapter digs into the competing ideologies surrounding risk that women, as the usual household decision makers about body and wellness issues, must navigate. The dominant US health ideology, which I call the "*risk-avoidant*" paradigm, holds that no cost is too great to bear when it comes to promoting a child's well-being. This ideology can be seen across popular parenting advice media, and it was echoed in the views that many mothers shared with me. Yet some mothers I spoke to were unwilling—or unable—to bear all of the material and physical costs associated with the risk-avoidant approach, and they instead made calculated decisions about where and when their resources could be best spent: adopting an alternative approach that I term the "*risk-assessing*" paradigm. Though less popular than the "risk-avoidant" approach, the risk-assessing framework has its proponents among at least some healthcare providers and parenting advice writers. Critically, while the risk-assessing approach challenges some elements of the risk-avoidant orthodoxy—namely, that risks to children should be minimized above all else—both paradigms share a deeper underlying belief: the idea that good mothering ought to be guided by scientific expertise, also known as "scientific motherhood."[1]

In this chapter, I argue that while all women are held accountable for following the dominant risk-avoidant paradigm as they "do health" in their reproductive body projects, not all women who deviate from it are judged equally. Middle-to-upper-class mothers, especially white women, are more likely to receive the benefit of the doubt that they are making responsible, well-informed decisions about risk for their children; they are granted space to make the decisions that work best for their own families. Poor and working-class mothers, on the other hand, face greater skepticism and judgment if they deviate from the risk-avoidant approach and are less likely to receive support from health workers and other authority figures for their choices. These low-status mothers are twice disadvantaged: first, by the material constraints of their class position, which place certain preventive health technologies and services out of financial reach; and second, by the class cultural differences that make it harder for these mothers to communicate their decision making in terms that healthcare providers will view as legitimate. Ultimately, while all mothers are likely to face occasional judgment for their choices as they are held accountable for doing health—and all will at least occasionally make compromises in the name of convenience or comfort—class and racial/ethnic differences mediate the potential social consequences they will face for these choices.

## "My body doesn't belong to me": Risk-Avoidant Motherhood

Although some mothers in this study found the work of navigating health choices during and after pregnancy rewarding, most cited a desire to avoid as many actual and potential health risks as possible as their overriding motivation. Indeed, the primary unifying theme among the diverse women I interviewed was the shared mission to protect children from harm. However, multiple harm-reduction strategies appeared among mothers. These strategies echoed the competing discourses present in wider US popular culture and society: Should mothers seek to minimize all risks to their children, no matter the size of the risk or the impact on mothers' own comfort and well-being? Or can they be trusted to take calculated risks, weighing the health benefits or costs of a choice alongside its other effects on themselves or their households?

Mixed-class Annie Castro (white, twenty-nine, HL), describing the many changes she made to her body-care regimen during pregnancy, summarized her outlook as follows: "If I can control something, I will. . . .

If there's an ounce [of a product] they're not really sure about, I just don't even do it. I can give up anything for my children and gladly do it."

With these words, Annie exemplifies the first of two strategies for managing risk, which I term "risk avoidant." This view holds that mothers should avoid anything that might possibly harm a baby, no matter how small the risk might be. Parenthood, especially as children get older, typically involves weighing trade-offs among safety, developmental opportunities, and convenience. During pregnancy and the postpartum period, however, many people hold the view that mothers can—and should—control everything in their child's environment and nutrition. Yet not all risks to pregnant people and fetuses have been scientifically evaluated: many common prescription drugs, for example, have not been tested for safety in pregnancy via controlled studies in humans; because fetal development is seen as particularly vulnerable, such studies may sometimes run afoul of scientific ethics. Similar issues exist for everyday household products and chemical additives that have neither been demonstrated to be safe nor definitively shown to be harmful in pregnancy. Potential risks associated with some of these drugs and chemicals may include miscarriage, prematurity, low birth weight, and teratogenicity (causing abnormalities in fetal development). In the absence of concrete evidence one way or another, women must make their own risk assessments, alone or (as in the case with pharmaceuticals) in consultation with their doctors. Many pregnant people and mothers engage in what Norah MacKendrick calls "precautionary consumption," using personal consumer choices as a way to mitigate against the hazards of living in a chemically risky environment.[2] The mindset behind this very individualized approach to risk avoidance is, as MacKendrick titles her book, "better safe than sorry."

Theresa Butler (white, thirty-three, HH) recounted seeing these views on the popular parenting websites she visited—BabyCenter and What to Expect—when she found out she was pregnant. "There's so many rules. It's ridiculous. Finding out [the rules] is easy, following it is hard because there is so much information. I can't keep all this shit in my head. . . . Like, you're not supposed to take ibuprofen while you're pregnant, right? Only acetaminophen? And I managed to switch that when I got pregnant with Isobel, so I was only taking ibuprofen. . . . It was all totally fine.

All these things they tell you not to do is because there's like one one-hundredth of a percent chance that something really bad might happen."

Advice against using ibuprofen-based pain relievers is based on research suggesting that ibuprofen use is associated with elevated risks of miscarriage or problems with fetal heart and lung development. Nevertheless, many other health recommendations are based on less conclusive evidence, and Theresa pointed out that the sheer *number* of "rules" for pregnancy health makes it easy for even conscientious mothers to get confused. Furthermore, the alarmist tone surrounding some of these guidelines—and the dire warnings about what could happen if they are not followed—left Theresa both surprised and relieved when her daughter was born perfectly healthy.

Like Theresa, mixed-class Cass Blackwell (white, thirty-three, LH) described the way she felt reading popular, risk-avoidant mothering advice magazines: "I've got subscriptions to a few magazines like *Self* and *Health*. And that was all stuff I was reading before [my daughter] came along. And now that she's here, I don't really have the time to devote to 'em. Maybe every so often I get a couple baby magazines that I try to read through, but I've determined that their main purpose in the world is to make every mother feel like she's doing it wrong. So I decided maybe I'll just stop reading them!" Cass continued, describing the advice she had recently gotten about the "healthier" way to mix formula:

> I was reading something the other day about formula and how shaking the formula, when you're mixing it, you lose nutrients, and that you should be stirring it. It's like, when you have a screaming baby, nobody's got time to stand there and *stir* [in mock-serious voice] the formula. This stuff is so clumpy, you have to shake the hell out of it to get it to mix up. So I just read that, and I was like, "Oh, there's one more thing for me to add to the list of things that I'm doing wrong, according to the book."

For Cass, risk-avoidant advice often had the effect of making her feel she was "doing it wrong"—she tried to take good care of her child, but it felt impossible to stay on top of so many parenting rules. Yet, while Cass and Theresa described the seemingly endless lists of health dos and don'ts as stressful and contrary to common sense, others described the same sets of dictates as somewhat helpful. Such was the case for Misty Clifford (white, thirty-one, HH), who admitted to following risk-avoidant approaches even though she did not know the details behind health recommendations: "I couldn't take prenatal vitamins, so I took Flintstones vitamins. And then it was like 'Oh, you should take folic acid when you're trying to get pregnant.' 'When you're breastfeeding, take extra DHA because it will help with brain development.' I don't know about all of that, the science of it. But it can't hurt, so why not?" Meanwhile, registered nurse Amanda Katz (white, thirty, HH) elaborated on her preference for organic foods, explaining, "I like to reduce the amount of pesticides that we ingest. You're sort of inundated with toxins, just walking around—car exhaust fumes and pollution. The problem is that we don't quite know what these pesticides are going to do to us in the long-term sense. So it seems prudent to try to reduce them as much as possible."

Amanda's cautious approach to risk ("We don't know what these pesticides are going to do to us . . . so it seems prudent to try to reduce them") and Misty's conclusion that "it [taking vitamins] can't hurt, so why not?" were typical of many middle- and upper-class women's accounts of their health choices. Even when these women did not understand the scientific evidence to support certain health practices—or when such evidence was scant—women with time and money to spare often poured their energies into these projects in hopes of securing at least some health and developmental advantages for their children. Similar to Annie Castro's statement that "I can give up anything for my children and gladly do it," Misty's statement that "it can't hurt" treats child well-being as an infinitely valuable good, worth any and all efforts and sacrifices new and expectant parents might invest. Building on the notion that children are now treated as "priceless,"[3] the risk-avoidant paradigm calls for constant investment in child well-being. I asked Misty where she had gathered these pieces of advice, to which she replied, "Doctors. Baby Center emails, or the 'What to Expect' book. Friends. And then the worst is the tribal knowledge with moms. I remember my mom and my mother-in-law and my grandmothers telling me you should do this and you shouldn't do that." Misty's rattling off of official, informal, and familial sources—the "tribal knowledge" of mothers—speaks to the ubiquity of the risk-avoidant paradigm.

The risk-avoidant approach also shows up in popular and government-sponsored materials promoting breastfeeding. During my fieldwork at WIC offices in Northern California, nutritionists handed out pamphlets extolling the benefits of breastmilk over commercial infant formula: "Compared to mother's breastmilk, formula is missing many things babies need to be strong, healthy, and smart. Did you know: formula-fed babies have a greater risk of ear infections, diarrhea/constipation, pneumonia, [and] SIDS (Sudden Infant Death Syndrome). Children who were formula-fed have a greater risk of: obesity (becoming overweight), diabetes, asthma and allergies, [and] cancer. *Formula feeding costs money . . . but the real cost of formula is the cost to your baby's health*" (emphasis added). This advice mirrored recommendations from the AAP and other health organizations at the time that "breast is best," asserting that breastmilk was a vastly superior choice for infant health and urging mothers to exclusively breastfeed for the first six months of a child's life. Subsequent studies have argued that these recommendations overstate the proven health benefits of breastmilk; the better health outcomes among breastfed babies appear, in many cases, to be due to the fact that those babies were born into families with economic and racial privilege.[4] Indeed, women who breastfeed are likely to be older, wealthier, and better educated relative to women who do not breastfeed.[5] In addition to these cultural trends that favor middle-class women's breastfeeding, practical and material considerations also make breastfeeding more likely among this group. Bernice Hausman explains, "Breastfeeding . . . is an activity facilitated by flexible work, social and financial resources, and supportive professional and kin networks."[6]

Nevertheless, at the time of this book's writing, the AAP and the National Institutes of Health (NIH) continued to recommend exclusive breastfeeding as the healthiest option for feeding infants, and WIC heavily promoted breastfeeding for participants.[7] In effect, recommendations such as those quoted above assert that *not* breastfeeding carries a risk—a risk of ear infections, diarrhea, pneumonia, and death, among other things—and urge mothers to avoid that risk by breastfeeding, regardless of how difficult it might be for some.

Mixed-class Noura Berry (white, twenty-three, HL) embraced this perspective on breastfeeding. Describing how she would advise another mother to breastfeed, she said, "It's for intelligence, personality. I mean, this is the best thing you can give your baby, and formula is just so artificial. . . . Even in the worst-case scenario, where it hurts like hell (like it did for me), I'm so grateful that I kept through it." Noura recounted significant pain during her early weeks of breastfeeding, but she felt that the potential benefits of breastfeeding to her son outweighed any temporary discomfort or inconvenience to herself. This view was shared by many other women I spoke to. Cass Blackwell described the litany of changes she made to her body-care practices during pregnancy:

> Even with colds, I didn't want to take medications or anything like that. I just wanted to do the best I possibly could for her. I have to take allergy medicine every day, which caused me all amounts of concern and worry, wondering if that was somehow going to affect her. I didn't dye my hair anymore. . . . For me, it was just a no-brainer. I read up about the foods I should be eating, took my prenatal vitamin religiously, completely avoided Cokes, even though I was dying to have one some days because I was so tired in the first trimester. But to me, it was easy: it's her that I have to be concerned about, not me. *My body doesn't belong to me during these nine months.* (emphasis added)

Cass, like Noura, did not find all of the changes she made *physically* easy. Even as her first-trimester fatigue often caused her to crave caffeine, she scrupulously resisted satisfying her cravings because of concerns about possible risks to her child. But for both Cass and Noura, the choice to put their child's needs above their own was *morally* easy. They reasoned that it was their duty, as expectant mothers, to make sacrifices to avoid any potential risks to their children.

Indeed, the widespread rituals of giving up caffeine and alcohol, avoiding taboo foods, and otherwise modifying self-care routines during pregnancy that so many women in my study described may serve an important role in socializing women into an ideal of self-sacrificing motherhood. As Charlotte Moran (biracial, thirty-two, HH) put it, "It was somewhat hard to give up coffee—that was the hardest thing. The other stuff [I gave up] was more of a bummer than anything, but mostly it was kind of fun preparation for having a baby. I kind of felt like I should be doing some kind of work! I should be doing something to get ready for this, and not just my body doing its thing!"

For Charlotte, as for many other women, the child-first, risk-avoidant approach to health during pregnancy often brought a mixture of emotions to first-time mothers: mild annoyance at the things they were missing out on (which Charlotte called "a bummer"); excitement as the changes helped make a mostly abstract notion of a future baby feel more real; and, as Cass noted, anxiety over whether they were doing enough to ensure their child's health. And while many women described pregnancy as a time for becoming particularly conscientious—as when Cass explained that "my body doesn't belong to me during those nine months"—this risk-avoidant attitude, and the child-first mindset it entailed, usually did not end at birth. Instead, as mother of eight Dawn Slade (white, thirty-three, LL) put it, "Between the house and the kids, you know, my children are my main priority over myself, so they always seem to come first." In other words, the child-health-centered mentality that mothers-to-be adopted during pregnancy was one that carried over into children's infancy and beyond.

To be clear, parents of all genders work and make sacrifices to promote their children's well-being. But just as Pierre Bourdieu observed in working-class families in twentieth-century France, Dawn's and other women's stories reveal a gendered expectation of the *ways* in which women will sacrifice their bodies' needs and comforts to care for children's (and male partners') physical well-being. Writing about households where food and other resources are scarce, Bourdieu explained that mothers are often the first to skip meals or limit their portions to ensure that others have enough to eat; he concludes, "A girl's accession to womanhood is marked by doing without."[8] In the present-day United States, the risk-avoidant perspective can be encapsulated by a reformulation of Bourdieu's words: a woman's accession to motherhood is marked by doing without caffeine, alcohol, sushi, and anything else that might pose a risk to her future children.

Women rarely specified the exact nature of the negative health outcomes they sought to avoid by avoiding risk. For example, some research suggests that consuming large quantities of caffeine during pregnancy can lead to lower birth weights (which, in turn, is associated with increased chances of certain health problems later in a child's life); but women I spoke to, and many of the advice sources they cited, did not address that specific outcome by name.[9] Rather, caffeine (and raw fish, unpasteurized cheese, "toxins," "chemicals," and a host of other substances) fell under a broad umbrella of risk: just don't do it.

In summary, the risk-avoidant perspective treats mothers' and children's bodies as linked. It urges women to make healthful choices on their children's behalf both during and after pregnancy, and holds that women's health will often benefit at the same time as their children's (such as through the adoption of a nutritious diet or regular exercise). And many women noted to me that they never took better care of their bodies than when they were pregnant or breastfeeding. Yet the risk-avoidant perspective also suggests that, when a conflict does arise between mothers' and babies' health and comfort, mothers' needs should come second: no price is too great to pay if it potentially benefits a child's health and development.

## "I did my research, and I thought it was okay": Risk-Assessing Motherhood

A second approach to making health decisions during and after pregnancy showed up among a handful of mothers I spoke to; I call this the "risk-assessing" approach. Lucy Wolff (white, thirty-three, HH) offered an example of this approach when she described a disagreement she had with her husband during her pregnancy: "My husband really wanted me to give up coffee and I'm like, 'Well, I really don't [want to]. So what are the risks?' And I looked up the studies, and found out that there really isn't that much risk to drinking a moderate amount of coffee."

Lucy's husband fell solidly into the risk-avoidant paradigm: he had heard that caffeine consumption during pregnancy might be bad for the baby, and he believed that the responsible choice was for Lucy to forego all caffeine to eliminate that risk. Lucy, however, pushed back; after doing some online reading about the evidence for avoiding coffee, she *assessed* her risk and determined that her current consumption habits were unlikely to affect her pregnancy. In another disagreement—this time over Lucy's practice of riding her bike to work while pregnant—Lucy defended her choices by saying, "I point out that driving a car is also dangerous, and that I'm a cautious bike rider and that the route is safe. . . . I just kind of calm his fears as much as I can. He's worried that somebody is going to hit me. Well, you know, that's a risk. But you can't just stay in your house and never go anywhere and never take a risk."

Whereas the risk-avoidant paradigm holds that any risk should be minimized—and that no cost is too great to bear if it can improve a child's chances for good health—the risk-assessing perspective instead accepts that most activities and types of consumption carry some degree of risk. The responsible mother, in this latter perspective, should educate herself about the particular risks of her choices and environment and make informed decisions on that basis. And while this approach still places a disproportionate burden on women to become health conscious, it also concedes that women are people who have the right to make choices to satisfy their own needs and comfort, not just ensure the well-being of their babies.

The risk-avoidant paradigm has long dominated—and, indeed, continues to dominate—the advice given to pregnant and postpartum women. Nevertheless, some women's doctors, midwives, and family members quietly offered alternative advice. For example, mixed-class Dani Hahn (white, twenty-four, LH) encountered two competing sets of advice about bed sharing: "I do hear a lot of 'You shouldn't be sleeping with your baby in your bed!' I get that from doctors, I get that from WIC. But at the same time, you'll see pediatric studies released about how [bed sharing] is actually better, because you can be closer to your baby. . . . My pediatrician says the things she has to say, and then she'll say, 'But off the record, I did it [shared a bed] with my kids, so *shhh*.' You know, they have to say what they have to say."

Dani's doctors and WIC counselors hewed to the official, risk-avoidant stance that bed sharing was dangerous (on the grounds that infants can suffocate or roll off the bed).[10] Yet as her pediatrician admitted, even health professionals sometimes broke these rules; for lactating mothers and colicky babies, bed sharing had the potential to promote the breastfeeding relationship and improve sleep for both parents and children. Parents who shared a bed with their babies were typically aware of the potential risks, but they addressed these risks by looking at the available research and, on the basis of that research, taking safety precautions like putting the mattress on the floor and removing loose bedding and pillows. And some health providers and WIC staff had begun to take a harm-reduction approach to bed sharing and other issues: officially counseling against the practice, while also providing information about how to do it as safely as possible.

In 2013, the risk-assessing approach to pregnancy found its champion in economist Emily Oster, whose popular book, *Expecting Better*, dug into the science behind common pregnancy health recommendations: its name not-so-subtly positions it as a counterpoint to the bestselling, risk-avoidant *What to Expect When You're Expecting*. Oster explains her data-driven approach: "[This book offers] the pregnancy numbers—the data to help [women] make their personalized pregnancy decisions and to help them understand their pregnancies in the clearest possible way, by the numbers. . . . We are often not given the opportunity to think critically about the decisions we make. Instead, we are expected to follow a largely arbitrary script without question. It's time to take control."[11]

Oster is neither the first nor the last to advocate that patients (and women in particular) should be given accurate information about their bodies and health options: for example, the women's health movement of the 1970s worked hard to demystify menstruation, childbirth, sexuality, and other issues in women's lives through educational workshops and publications.[12] And during the COVID-19 pandemic that hit the United States in 2020, Oster was joined by public health experts like Dr. Katelyn Jetelina (blogging at *Your Local Epidemiologist*) and physicians Ashish Jha and Leana Wen (frequent contributors in the *New York Times* and *Washington Post*, and parents of young children as well), all of whom offered families advice for assessing their health risks in the face of rapidly developing information about this deadly new illness.[13] Rather than advocating one-size-fits-all prescriptions for health, these experts acknowledged that different people's levels of risk tolerance and ability to avoid risk might vary significantly, and offered readers the tools to calculate their own risks accordingly. These risk assessments were particularly charged for parents, who had to weigh the uncertain health risks of COVID infection in young children (and in anyone those children might infect) against the costs of keeping children home (costs that included impacts on parents' careers, children's schooling, and children's social development). Oster's assertion that mothers need better information on which to base their decisions thus represents one especially prominent example of the broader risk-assessing approach to health.

In the years since its publication, Oster's work has been profoundly polarizing, drawing both praise and scorn from parents and public health experts alike. Many readers—whom Oster describes as "coastal-dwelling, college-educated people who like numbers and are 'probably fairly anxious'"—welcomed the perspective that they could be trusted to make informed decisions for their families: that they could *assess risks* responsibly.[14] Others hammered Oster for her permissiveness. In the Amazon reviews for the book, reviewer "Amazonian Queen" concluded, "If you'd like someone to make you feel like it's fine to drink alcohol during your pregnancy, this book may be for you. But if you're serious about learning and making the safest choices for you and your baby, look elsewhere."[15] Likewise, commenter "T. Freeborn" added, "I just think having a baby is the time to get a little selfless and giving up a few things even if it MAY give your baby a better chance is worth it."[16] Such comments neatly illustrate the risk-avoidant perspective, assuming that all pregnant people—at least all who are responsible—would prefer to minimize all risks to their babies, no matter the likelihood or severity of those risks.

To be clear, women who adopted a risk-assessing stance were rarely antimedicine. They valued medical knowledge when it came to their most pressing health concerns, but they rejected the notion that they should unthinkingly give up all of their comforts when they became pregnant. Such was the case for Chevonne Lewis (Black, twenty-three, LL), who was prescribed a restrictive diet when she developed gestational diabetes. She followed her doctor's instructions on limiting sugary foods but gave herself permission to continue drinking sugar-free soda, saying, "The doctor told me that the equivalent of one cup of coffee was okay. And I did my research, and I thought it was okay. I drank as much Diet Coke as I wanted . . . because it didn't have anything in it!"

Chevonne recounted how strangers would chide her for drinking soda, and explained, "I'd just let people talk until they were finished and then say thank you. I did think about what they said, but I didn't really do things differently." Although risk-assessing mothers did not always defend their choices to would-be advice givers, they often seethed with frustration when observers chimed in. Most risk assessors described their decisions as based in their extensive experience or information gathering, but when they got risk-avoidant advice, they felt that the subtext to the comments was that they were either ignorant or willfully disregarding children's health—in any case, that they were bad mothers.

Stories like the ones above highlight the contradictions between the risk-avoidant and risk-assessing paradigms: risk avoidance was the dominant stance adopted by mothers and advice givers alike, and those who opted for risk assessment often felt the need to defend their choices to the risk avoiders. But while the risk-assessing framework challenges certain assumptions of the risk-avoidant perspective—chiefly through its belief that risk is calculable, and that some level of risk is acceptable and unavoidable—both paradigms share a deeper underlying foundation. Critically, both uphold elements of "scientific motherhood," which is the "belief that women require expert scientific and medical advice to raise their children healthfully."[17] Perhaps, rather than as two entirely distinct or opposed paradigms, it is more helpful to view them as two branches of scientific motherhood: one that sees women primarily as passive recipients of scientific and medical advice (risk avoidant), and one that expects women to act as informed, active consumers of expert knowledge (risk assessing). In the former, the roles of experts and mothers are distinct: scientific and medical professionals teach mothers about health risks, and mothers then follow their guidance. In the latter, responsible mothers do not merely receive advice but are empowered to sift through conflicting advice to oversee the health of their families and to exercise their own discretion, provided their choices are grounded in scientific evidence.

The risk-assessing perspective's basis in scientific and medical expertise enables its practitioners to assert their status as good mothers. This also means it is more accessible to middle- and upper-class mothers, or at least those who are highly educated. As I will discuss in chapter 4, numerous poor and working-class women express ambivalence about hegemonic health and body-care standards generally, and the ideology of risk avoidance specifically. But while a handful of lower-income women deploy risk-assessing rhetoric to explain their choices, the majority draw on alternative cultural repertoires: behaviors and accounts that reflect their own best judgment about how to care for themselves and their children, but that are less likely to be legible to health authorities as evidence of "good" scientific motherhood.

Ultimately, the risk-avoidant and risk-assessing approaches to maternal embodiment and wellness start from the premise that women's body-care choices, at least during pregnancy and for some time thereafter, make a difference in their children's health and development. The risk-avoidant perspective, which predominates in official advice to mothers as well as in the views women themselves held, is rooted in gendered notions of appropriate femininity as nurturing, selfless, and unconditionally attuned to others' needs. Pregnancy and breastfeeding are the times most commonly targeted for modifying women's body-care and consumption practices, due to the porous connections between mothers' and children's bodies (and thus they are the times when mothers' habits pose the greatest risk or opportunity to their children). Yet, I argue, these stages also socialize women into an ethos of self-sacrificing motherhood that extends far beyond the postpartum period. The risk-assessing perspective, in contrast, offers women the "opportunity to think critically about the decisions [they] make" (as Oster puts it) and to decide for themselves which sacrifices seem worthwhile. On one hand, the risk-assessing perspective accords women some agency and recognizes that their needs, tastes, and preferences may be weighed alongside health risks to children. On the other hand, women who assessed their risks and decided, for example, that drinking coffee during pregnancy or opting not to breastfeed was the best option for them were often forced to justify their choices to others. Their approaches to defending their choices—and their legibility as good mothers—were, I argue, patterned by class.

## When Some Costs Are Too Great: Class as Material Inequality

As the previous chapter explained, during and after pregnancy women shoulder a disproportionate weight of responsibility for children's health and well-being. This burden often rests on a foundation of women's own body consciousness that was laid long before they became mothers, wherein they became conversant in the language of dieting, nutrition, delayed gratification, and other ways of "doing health." Once they have children, these women learn to extend their body consciousness to the family members they care for, noticing and responding to everyday bodily needs and looking ahead to long-term developmental arcs. A good mother, in this system, must both educate herself about the health risks and benefits of particular body-care practices and make choices in line with what she has learned; fathers tended to take on the role of well-intentioned—but often clueless—"helpers." During pregnancy and breastfeeding especially, the dominant risk-avoidant discourse holds that no cost or inconvenience to mothers is too great if it might minimize a child's risk of harm. This section and the next look at the implications of this "no cost is too great" risk-avoidant mindset for women of limited means, as well as the class dynamics of the alternative "risk-assessing" approach to body care.

For households with different incomes, the risk-avoidant position that no cost is too great represents vastly different impacts on household budgets. For example, a number of middle- and upper-class women in my study described breastfeeding as a necessary risk-prevention strategy, even though many of the purported benefits of breastmilk remain unproven or relatively minor. When Emily Fischer (white, thirty-one, HH) was nursing her infant, she developed a two-month bout of thrush (a yeast infection that can cause pain in breastfeeding and be transmitted back and forth between the breast and the infant's mouth) that hastened her decision to stop nursing. Hesitant to offer formula—and convinced of the benefits of breastmilk—Emily and her husband considered purchasing donor milk at the cost of $4.50 an ounce. Given that a typical six-month-old might drink thirty-two ounces of milk a day, feeding their child donor milk exclusively would have cost over a thousand dollars *per week*. For Emily, as well as many other high-status mothers I interviewed, the potential but uncertain benefits of breastmilk—and the risks it might protect against—were worth significant time, money, and emotional investment.

Not all women had the flexible jobs, time, or financial resources to make these kinds of choices. Nicole Johnson (Black, twenty-two, LL) was eager to breastfeed when she became pregnant, explaining, "I always knew I would breastfeed. My mom breastfed all of us, so that wasn't a problem. All of us [my cousins and I] had our kids around the same time. Everyone else was like, 'We're not going to do it because it hurts.' But I'm a tough person, so you can't tell me something like that." Nicole followed through on her plan and managed to breastfeed her daughter Keshia for eight months. Lactation consultants at WIC urged her to breastfeed for a full year but, she explained, "I was working all different hours, so it was hard and I wasn't pumping enough milk. They weren't understanding that it's not enough for Keshia and then I would have to leave work early. I had to change over [to formula]; it just wasn't working out."

Nicole was well educated about the benefits of breastmilk and, like many middle-class respondents, she made a plan to breastfeed for at least the first year of her child's life. Unlike these women's, though, Nicole's plan came into conflict with financial and workplace constraints: keeping her job meant following an unpredictable work schedule, which made it difficult to pump and maintain a supply for Keshia when she was not home. For Nicole, the potential, uncertain benefits of breastfeeding her daughter for four more months were outweighed by the immediate benefits of holding down a full-time job and financially supporting her family.

Jazmine Easton (Black, thirty-four, LL), a mother of five, felt that breastfeeding was a luxury only stay-at-home mothers could afford; for women like Jazmine—who often spent hours every day on public transit or in the waiting rooms of public service agencies—nursing and pumping seemed utterly impractical. As she put it, "Every individual, it's different. It depends on what you [do for] work and school. If you on the go and moving, it's impossible. . . . I ain't fixin' to be at the bus stop, going 'Here, baby.'" As she said this, Jazmine chuckled and mimed cradling a baby to her breast with one arm, grabbing an overhead strap with the other. Although Jazmine allowed that some women did make this arrangement work, she concluded, "I couldn't." Jazmine's doubts about how breastfeeding could fit into her busy days and lack of privacy illustrate what a growing number of cultural commentators have noted in recent years: the common refrain of breastfeeding advocates—that breastmilk is free—is only true if we believe that women's time has no value.[18] This position assumes that the time women spend breastfeeding—often several hours a day—is not time they could be spending earning money or engaged in other productive activities.

Beyond breastfeeding, mothers noted other financial challenges they faced in nourishing their children's (and their own) bodies. In many cases, they tried to meet the demands of "precautionary consumption,"[19] which urges mothers to avoid pesticides and other harmful chemicals by opting for organic products. Yet eating that way is costly. MacKenzie Gervais (white, thirty, HH) described her family's meals thus: "Most lunches and dinners include some sort of a meat for us, unless it's spaghetti night. . . . We'll have spaghetti night just because I'm not going to buy the crappy ground beef, and we can't afford five nights of lean organic chicken."

For middle-class mothers like MacKenzie, the imperative to eat high-quality food was so strong that she would rather go without meat at one or more meals than serve her children "crappy ground beef." Mixed- and working-class mothers who received WIC benefits, meanwhile, often spoke with frustration about the program's prohibition on using WIC checks for organic foods; they had absorbed the popular message that organic food was best for their children, and did not understand why a government program supposedly dedicated to improving maternal and child health would deny them what they believed to be the most health-ful option.

All mothers faced some cost that was too great—a health-promoting product or practice that was beyond their family's time or financial means. But mixed-class mothers, especially those with middle-class cul-tural references but a working-class budget, exemplified the pain of the "no cost is too great" mindset most acutely.

Gita Potter (Asian, twenty-seven, HL), a mixed-class mother who stayed home with her child while her husband, a medical student, at-tended school, explained, "In an ideal world, I'd have more money, and that would free up resources to be able to spend money on better-quality things. I would love to be able to shop at Trader Joe's instead of the Grocery Outlet for produce, or to get better-quality peaches. But that's not really in the budget right now." Gita's agonizing over the costs of fresh produce was a common refrain among mixed-class mothers. Christine Webber (white, thirty-seven, HL) had experienced significant financial upheaval over the previous several years, during which time she had earned two master's degrees (but also become dependent on public benefits). And, during that time, she had learned to use food as a measure of her household's financial well-being: "If there's fresh fruit in the house, even if it's just some bananas in the bowl or some apples or something, then I really feel like, 'We're doing alright now.' Because that, to me, seems expensive and immediately perishable, so you actu-ally have to move through it kind of fast. If it's there, then you must be doing pretty good."

Like Christine and Gita, Nicki Lindsay (white, thirty, HL) believed in the health value of eating fresh produce even as she struggled to af-ford it. When funds were tight, she—embracing the child-first ethos of the risk-avoidant approach—fed her children vegetables while forgoing them herself. She started to explain this choice as her own failure to eat healthily, but added, "You know, we have a food budget. So I want to save the best stuff for them. That's part of it." Mixed-class Noura Berry (white, twenty-three, HL) was an avid practitioner of attachment parenting and elimination communication: parenting practices popular among mostly class-privileged mothers that emphasize, respectively, near-constant physical contact between a parent and baby, and diaperless toileting for infants and toddlers (wherein caregivers learn to interpret a baby's physical signs of an impending need to urinate or defecate).[20] Noura spoke longingly of the top-of-the-line Ergobaby backpack-style carrier she wished she could afford for her solidly built son. Lacking that carrier, she often transported her heavy baby in her arms, but it was uncomfortable. She added, "People who have my level of poverty [usually] shop at the dollar store for their clothes and eat Fruit Loops, but I don't. You know, my financial level doesn't reflect my habitus."

Noura's comments reveal her simultaneous identification with more highly educated women (such as in her use of "habitus," a term from French social theory, to describe her cultural class) and her efforts to distinguish herself from her socioeconomic peers. Throughout our interview, Noura repeatedly drew symbolic boundaries between herself and the other women who occupied her financial status, claiming higher moral and cultural prestige on the basis of her parenting knowledge and desired consumption patterns. Not all mixed-class mothers drew such stark divisions between themselves and others, but their position between classes—which often meant they had cultural access to the norms for middle-class parenting but not the financial means to achieve these norms—made them particularly sensitive to the material demands of risk-avoidant motherhood.

The "no cost is too great" mindset of the risk-avoidant paradigm requires mothers to sacrifice their time, comfort, and financial resources on behalf of their children's health and well-being, sacrifices fathers are rarely asked to make. Yet, as these mothers' stories show, expenditures that represent a manageable expense for some women (e.g., exclusive breastfeeding, eating organic) remain utterly out of reach for others. What are the consequences of this disparity for mothers' ability to see themselves—and be seen by others—as good mothers? And while *all* mothers must sometimes assess risks and make compromises—to save money or time, or in the face of conflicting advice—which mothers are viewed as responsible enough to make such choices?

## One Glass of Wine: Class as Cultural Inequality

As the earlier discussion of risk-assessing approaches illustrates, women across classes occasionally felt the need to compromise or make adjustments to the official recommendations for body care during and after pregnancy. Whether it was Lucy Wolff's insistence that scientific research supported her one-cup-a-day coffee habit during pregnancy or Dani Hahn's belief that the sleep and breastfeeding benefits of bed sharing with her infant outweighed the risks, mothers from different class backgrounds at least occasionally made the determination that some warnings about risk were being overstated. In other words, even though the risk-avoidant paradigm dominated popular discourse, in practice, everyone engaged in risk assessment from time to time. The degree to which mothers were *trusted* to make these determinations, however, was not evenly distributed. Describing the changing cultural attitudes toward mothers' infant-feeding choices, Linda Blum writes, "If today we have learned to trust *some* women's bodies, it is only those of the proper race and class, not to mention marital status, age, and sexual orientation" (emphasis in original).[21] Indeed, women in my study who diverged from the risk-avoidant stance faced significantly different levels of trust from their medical providers and other sources of health advice, largely tied to class.

Nowhere is the classing of trust more evident than in providers' advice about alcohol consumption. In its 2015 statement on prenatal alcohol use, the American Academy of Pediatrics (AAP) asserted, "Although a consensus is still lacking about the effects of low levels of PAE [prenatal alcohol exposure], harmful effects are well documented related to moderate or greater PAE and to binge drinking. . . . The healthiest choice regarding alcohol use during pregnancy is to abstain."[22] The AAP's stance is based on the reasoning that because higher levels of alcohol intake have proven risks, any level of drinking should be considered risky. In 2016, the CDC went even further in its recommendations, stating that because many people do not know they are pregnant until several weeks after conception, anyone who might *potentially* be pregnant should abstain from alcohol use. This recommendation expands the risk-avoidant approach beyond pregnancy to include the majority of (hetero)sexually active women of childbearing age, no matter how likely or desired pregnancy might be for them.

I did not ask women directly about drinking while pregnant; however, in response to my open-ended question about changes women made during pregnancy, nine mothers volunteered that they drank—at least a little bit—during pregnancy. They did so in direct contradiction to the AAP's stance on alcohol in pregnancy, though not, as it happened, in contradiction to their healthcare providers.

Stephanie Brewer (white, thirty-two, HH) recalled, "My gynecologist prescribed me red wine when I was overdue [to give birth]. He was like, 'You're supposed to drink a glass of wine every night. Go get a massage, go get a pedicure.'" Given that Stephanie's general attitude toward pregnancy was that she wanted to have the "absolute perfect pregnancy," her doctor may have been reacting specifically to Stephanie's anxiety and perfectionism, hoping to alleviate some of her worry as she waited to go into labor. Yet Stephanie was not the only woman I interviewed who was advised to drink a glass of wine. Suzanne Walsh (white, thirty-five, HH) described her "super-moderate" obstetrician as having told her, "You can drink a glass of wine, eat what you want." Bree Turner (white, thirty-three, HH) told me her midwife had given Bree her blessing to drink a cup of coffee every day and, later in pregnancy, "to occasionally have a glass of wine." And mixed-class Cass Blackwell (white, thirty-three, LH) followed her doctor's advice even though it made her anxious: "I didn't drink at all, until maybe the final couple weeks, when I was just so uncomfortable. And the doctor pretty much said, 'Just have a glass of wine to relax.'"

Several other women told me that they preferred not to drink, but that they thought it would be fine if they did: Lori Kent (white, twenty-nine, HH) noted that "I had done some research on that, and even up to one drink on a full stomach" would be fine, and Miranda Hughes (white, thirty-six, HH) added, "I don't think drinking in moderation would be harmful during pregnancy," citing research that failed to show a link between moderate drinking and fetal alcohol syndrome. Other women, like Charlotte Moran (white, thirty-two, HH), would "occasionally have a glass of wine" on the basis of their own information gathering and the determinations they made about risk. Charlotte added that she valued having friends with whom she could drink her occasional glass of wine while pregnant, free from judgment.

There are several striking aspects to the ways these mothers spoke about their relationship to alcohol during pregnancy. First, every woman who discussed drinking—or even considering drinking—while pregnant used almost identical language: "one glass of wine." A handful of my respondents described abstaining from beer while they were pregnant, and one—Britta Larson—told a heart-wrenching story about having a beer while she was miscarrying and in pain; in that moment, she was not choosing to drink while pregnant but was drinking in recognition of the pregnancy's end. But for women and care providers who believed that women could drink responsibly while pregnant, the phrase that represented appropriate moderation was always "a glass of wine."

The symbolic meanings of wine matter here. On one hand, wine is seen as "classy"—an often-expensive marker of taste, intended to be consumed alongside a meal instead of for the purpose of getting drunk. On the other hand, wine may also be feminized, so it is seen as a more appropriate drink for women than beer or hard alcohol.[23] More specifically, wine enjoys a reputation as being the drink of middle- and upper-class mothers (seen in the pop-cultural phenomenon of the suburban "wine mom" who sips a glass of white wine—or maybe several—in the evening to deal with the stress of being a wife and mother).[24] Whereas hard liquor and beer carry cultural connotations of excess, staying out late, and getting drunk, "a glass of wine" calls to mind civility and restraint: characteristics more in line with the idealized image of a good mother. Indeed, physicians and midwives who endorsed relaxing with a glass of wine late in pregnancy may have made this recommendation only to women they perceived as possessing these idealized traits of restraint and responsibility, or with the implicit aim of reinforcing the necessity of such traits.

Second, and relatedly, the "one glass of wine" mothers I spoke to were, almost entirely, white and middle to upper class (one woman, mixed-class Cass, was an upwardly mobile white woman from a working-class background; another, Charlotte, was the middle-class, light-skinned daughter of a Chinese American mother and Irish American father). Not one poor or working-class mother, and not one Black or Latina mother I interviewed ever recounted a medical provider telling them they could have a glass of wine.

In place of the permissive understanding that high-status white mothers often received from their providers, poor and working-class mothers were more likely to face scolding when they diverged from providers' understandings of best practices. For example, mixed-class Frankie Ford (white, twenty-six, LH) recounted adding rice cereal to her son's formula bottle earlier than is typically recommended. She told me that her WIC counselor "just scolded me for giving him all that stuff early." But Frankie felt that her son was not getting full from formula alone, and he also struggled with GERD (reflux) that caused him to vomit when she offered him unaltered liquid formula. She explained how, paying careful attention to her son's body, she adjusted his diet: "When he was a few weeks old I started putting in the rice [cereal], just a half teaspoon, maybe, to thicken it up a little bit. And he was puking less, so I moved it up from half a teaspoon to a full teaspoon, and he stopped puking altogether. I got in trouble for that [at WIC], but I still did it."

In many ways, Frankie's story epitomizes the careful attention that society expects mothers to cultivate. She noted her son's special needs and, taking sole responsibility for his care, made dietary changes that she believed would make him healthier and more comfortable. Nevertheless, Frankie "got in trouble" for going against her care providers' advice. Worth noting is that the AAP, citing an article from its flagship journal, *Pediatrics*, actually backs Frankie's approach: "The feeding management strategy that involves the use of thickened feedings, either by adding up to 1 tablespoon of dry rice cereal per 1 oz of formula or changing to commercially thickened (added rice) formulas for full-term infants who are not cow milk protein intolerant, is recognized as a reasonable management strategy for otherwise healthy infants with both GER and GERD."[25]

Many WIC counselors asserted to me that mothers in WIC chose formula over breastmilk, as well as sometimes thickening formula with rice cereal, because those options were harder to digest and caused babies to sleep longer. The implication of these claims was that such mothers were unwilling to do what was healthiest for their babies—breastfeeding—

because they selfishly wanted to sleep more. Whether or not this was the case for some women, the fact that counselors held this belief meant that they "scolded" Frankie (and other women) for adopting what the AAP calls a "reasonable management strategy" for infants with special needs like GERD. This treatment contrasts sharply with the trend, discussed above, wherein middle- and upper-class white pregnant women were granted permission to drink—again, in *opposition to* the AAP's directives—by care providers who perceived them to be responsible, moderate, good mothers.

Although wine and caffeine were the two most common "risky" substances women admitted to using during pregnancy, a handful of women spoke to me about additional substance use and other potential risks during the course of our interviews together. Lara Noble (white, forty, HH) recounted her fertility struggles after spending most of her twenties as a regular smoker and drinker who experimented with numerous other recreational drugs. Mixed-class Dani Hahn (white, twenty-four, LH) likewise had a history of smoking and drug use (including an arrest for narcotics possession in her late teens). And among poor and working-class white mothers, at least six described themselves as current or former smokers who struggled to quit or cut back during their pregnancies. Notably, not one Black or Latina participant volunteered a history of smoking or illicit drug use, but several spoke about the urgency they felt about keeping their children away from drugs.

These findings do not conclusively show which women smoked or used other drugs during pregnancy. I did not regularly ask about smoking and drug use, but rather relied on subjects to report on health behaviors and changes to their routines during and after pregnancy; these racial and class differences in reported behaviors may reflect actual differences in women's rates of using nicotine and other drugs, but they might also reflect the different levels of comfort women felt in admitting to these behaviors (and for good reason: white women are less likely than Black or Native women to be prosecuted or lose custody for alleged drug use or child endangerment).[26] Regardless of which explanation is correct, both reflect the same underlying phenomenon: women in welfare programs—Black and brown women especially—are at risk of being labeled as "bad mothers" for failing to adequately protect their children or set a good example. Low-income women of color are keenly aware of these stereotypes; knowing the added scrutiny they are likely to face, they may be more cautious about straying from the risk-avoidant paradigm (or, at the very least, more cautious about admitting to it). Thus, while the alternative risk-assessing approach for making health and body-care decisions offered women the chance to attend to their own needs from time to time, mothers who were not white and middle to upper class faced greater costs for deviating from the hegemonic risk-avoidant paradigm.

## Conclusion

This chapter explores the dominant and alternative approaches women in my study used for managing risks to their children's health. Respectively, these are the risk-avoidant paradigm, which views any avoidable risk to children as unacceptable (and prioritizes children's needs over mothers'), and the risk-assessing paradigm, in which women seek to balance risk management with other priorities like maternal health, comfort, and convenience. In the United States, the hegemony of the risk-avoidant paradigm means that all women are subject to judgment when they make body-care decisions that others perceive to be unnecessarily risky—or, at least, as inadequately focused on the healthist goal of bodily optimization.

Deborah Lupton explains that risk awareness is a critical part of contemporary health values more generally: "Risk [is] a consequence of the 'lifestyle' choices made by individuals, and thus places the emphasis on self-control. Individuals are exhorted by health promotion authorities to evaluate their risk of succumbing to disease and to change their behavior accordingly."[27] In this climate, pursuing health and avoiding risk is no longer a matter of personal preference but a moral responsibility of all good citizens. Those who have the will and ability to adopt practices in line with this expectation enjoy status benefits in addition to any tangible health benefits they might achieve.

The converse, that people who appear insufficiently invested in avoiding health risks will experience moral judgment, is also true. But that judgment is not experienced equally. A number of middle- and upper-class mothers I spoke to described practices that defied the tenets of modern risk-avoidant motherhood: drinking wine late in pregnancy, sometimes on the recommendation of their health provider; consuming caffeine; and histories of pre-pregnancy substance use that conflict with the demands of "anticipatory motherhood" that Miranda Waggoner describes.[28] Yet, as discussed in chapter 1, middle- and upper-class mothers were more likely to feel comfortable second-guessing or contradicting mainstream medical advice. Such women had both the educational and the professional backgrounds to seek out health information for themselves and the cultural status to assert their preferences with medical providers whom they saw as equals, rather than authority figures. And health providers were more likely to perceive class-privileged women as being, if anything, *too* health-conscious and to suggest they worry less about risks. For example, when then-pregnant Suzanne Walsh called her obstetrician in a panic because she ate a fish known to have higher levels of mercury, her doctor urged her not to worry, saying, "It's fine." And when Emily Fischer struggled through pain and infection to exclusively breastfeed her infant, she recounted that "even the lactation consultants were like, you know, you've gone above and beyond any mom we've ever met. You have permission to stop, and it's okay."

In contrast, poor and working-class mothers rarely, if ever, interacted with health providers and WIC staff who told them to worry less about risk. One main function of WIC consultations was to reinforce and build on low-income mothers' risk consciousness: raising concerns about child tooth decay, urging caregivers to limit portion sizes and high-calorie foods, pushing breastfeeding as the healthiest option, and more. To be clear, I do not assume that all discussions with parents about their children's health carry moral judgment. And given that health disparities often fall along socioeconomic lines in the United States, offering low-income families advice and material resources to access better nutrition, as WIC does, is a worthwhile goal.

But as this chapter's stories demonstrate, women in different classes experienced noticeably different interactions with health providers in relation to risk. Time and again, middle- and upper-class mothers encountered providers who trusted them and assumed that they were knowledgeable and responsible, even to the point of urging them to relax their risk-avoidant behaviors. In contrast, poor and working-class mothers faced interactions with WIC staff and other health professionals who wanted them to do more: to learn more about health and health risks and to incorporate that knowledge into their daily body-care practices. In the wider context of a culture that views the "risk-avoidant" paradigm as the most loving, responsible, morally righteous approach—and that describes risk-assessing mothers as selfish or worse—what might be the effects of these divergent classed experiences?

As Molly Ladd-Taylor and Lauri Umansky remind us, "The 'bad' mother label does not necessarily denote practices that actually harm children. In fact, it serves to shift our attention away from a specific act to a whole person—and even to entire categories of people. Thus doctors are far more likely to diagnose fetal alcohol syndrome in the child of a Native American than in the child of a WASP, [and] police and social workers are conditioned to look for juvenile delinquency among the sons of welfare mothers."[29] In the context of the present study, assumptions about who is sufficiently health conscious—and who is "at risk"—are only a short distance from judgments about who is a good or bad mother. Those assumptions, linked to race and class, may cause health providers to grant middle- and upper-class mothers, especially white women, the leeway to use their own discretion in health matters, while second-guessing poor or mixed-class women like Frankie Ford who made health choices that fit the needs of their family.

Lastly, while this chapter attends primarily to the disparate experiences that exist among women of different racial/ethnic and class identities, it bears repeating that moral debates over which mothers are sufficiently risk avoidant typically let fathers off the hook altogether. Reproductive body projects like nurturing a pregnancy or initiating and maintaining breastfeeding may strike us as being the sole responsibility of people with particular bodies: for the most part, mothers. But, as Cynthia Daniels explains, "Men's physical distance from gestation creates the illusion that men's relation to fetal health is tangential, [when] in reality a man's use of drugs or alcohol or his exposures to toxins long before conception can profoundly affect the health of the children he fathers."[30] And fathers' behaviors during and after a partner's pregnancy, such as smoking, can also increase or mitigate risk. In other words, moral discourses about risk avoidance and risk assessment take place in a larger social context that not only assumes certain women are more responsible than others but also scrutinizes women and their bodies while exempting men altogether.

# 4

## The Stories Mothers Tell

*Class Identity in Women's Body-Care Narratives*

Patrice Martin (Black, thirty-six, LL), a mother of four living in Florida, contrasted the tastes she was trying to cultivate in her children to her own, admittedly less nutritious preferences: "I try to get more fruits and vegetables. I'm not one of them kinds of people [who likes produce], but I at least want to try to raise them up on that. . . . I used to eat greens, but I don't eat them no more over the years. I will try to raise [my kids] . . . to like those foods. This is not what I like, but I'm just trying." Patrice made clear that she did not enjoy the fruits and vegetables that she perceived to constitute healthful eating. Nevertheless, she tried to get her children to eat fresh produce because she thought it was most nutritious for them, and she encouraged them to eat baked rather than fried foods.

In contrast, Joan Zimmerman (white, thirty-eight, HH), a Florida mother of two, was more permissive with her children's diets than with her own. Joan described herself as the "crunchy" daughter of an "earthy-crunchy-granola mom" who had taught her to grow and make many of her own foods.[1] Nowadays, she gave and received advice in a local attachment-parenting group made up of fellow "crunchy moms" devoted to studying a parenting style described by proponents as "intuitive."[2] Recently, Joan had adopted a diet that she learned of in that group and explored on her own: "I have investigated a new way of eating, and it's called primal eating. It's basically looking at how our ancestors, before we discovered agriculture, would have eaten: eating meat and nuts and vegetables and fruits, and staying away from grains and sugar, because that puts a large load on our bodies. I've found that that's actually a really good way for me to eat. I've lost about ten pounds doing it in the last month. I don't get hungry, and I don't crave things." Although Joan was new to the "primal eating" trend, she tied this latest diet to her more general identification as "crunchy" and health focused, her background of being raised by a mother who taught her to think about health, and her belief in the importance of seeking out information about health. She added, "Mothering.com has a forum on traditional eating, which I'm getting more and more interested in for my kids. Because at this point they're not going to give up grains. . . . But there are ways of preparing grains which are traditional and may help make them healthier and more digestible." Joan did not have acute concerns about her children's health that she was trying to solve through these dietary changes. Instead, she had come to believe that so-called primal eating was the better, more natural way to eat, and she was working to convert her husband and children to eating in this way, too.[3]

For Joan, as for many other middle- and upper-class mothers, cultivating a reproductive body project became a way to put her values into practice. Throughout our interview, Joan voiced strong opinions about health and body issues, ranging from the ingredients in allergy medication ("disgusting") to her postpartum body image ("I like being strong and I like being nourishing, I'm not crazy about my varicose veins"). Through her carefully chosen body-management practices and her stated rationales for how she made those choices, Joan used her reproductive body project to claim a particular self-identity ("crunchy," health-focused, and intentional). In contrast, Patrice and many other poor and working-class women resisted crafting self-identity narratives—or, at least, resisted tying their health and body-care practices to identity. Indeed, in her statement about disliking fresh produce, Patrice seemed to be *disidentifying* with the imperative to eat healthfully through consuming fruits and vegetables. That is, even as she tried to cultivate a taste for these foods in her children—and in so doing, acknowledged her belief that this was a better way to eat—she asserted her own tastes and preferences in opposition to the healthist norm that said not only that she should eat greens but also that she should like them.

This chapter looks at the processes of embodied identity construction and disidentification in which women engaged, both in their everyday body-care practices and in how they narrated those practices to me. While "identity" can seem very personal and individual, it is also a way of positioning oneself in relationship to broader social norms, groupings, and classifications that has consequences for social status. As I will show, mothers from different class backgrounds spoke about identity in distinct ways—with, I argue, divergent consequences for their ability to make status claims through that identity.

## Risk and Self-Identity

Joan's approach to investigating and enacting a particular reproductive body project—in this case, choosing "primal eating" for herself and working to introduce elements of that approach into her family's diet—neatly illustrates Anthony Giddens's account of late modern "body regimes" aimed at cultivating "self-identity." Echoing the themes of risk avoidance raised in chapter 3, Giddens explains, "Lifestyle choice is increasingly important in the constitution of self-identity and daily activity. Reflexively organized life-planning, which normally presumes consideration of risks as filtered through contact with expert knowledge, becomes a central feature of the structuring of identity."[4]

Put another way, a feature of early-twenty-first-century life in the West is the expectation that individuals will self-consciously adopt a *lifestyle*—an intentional approach to everyday living—that emphasizes understanding and managing one's risks. That lifestyle then becomes part of a coherent "self-identity" we cultivate for ourselves, which is "routinely created and sustained in the reflexive activities of the individual."[5] For Giddens, intentionally chosen actions, plus periodic reflection on the meaning of those activities, forms the basis for an individual's self-identity. Once again, Joan's lengthy discussion of her approach to health offers a useful illustration: "I used to call my mom earthy-crunchy-granola mom, because she used to bake her own bread and make her own yogurt and have things like lentil and barley stew and gross stuff. You know, it's funny, I'm turning into my mom! I'm not making my kids eat lentil and barley stew, but I bake my own bread. I think that good nutrition is really important, and over the years I've learned more about the high fructose corn syrup and the hydrogenated oils, and eating organic. And I learned about it from my mom."

In this telling, Joan's progression from childhood reluctance at eating "health" foods to "turning into my mom" becomes a narrative of healthy eating as her birthright, a legacy inherited from her mother. Furthermore, Joan's story features "reflexively organized life-planning" (making conscientious choices in light of long-term health goals) and the "consideration of risks as filtered through contact with expert knowledge" (knowledge about "risky" foods like high fructose corn syrup and hydrogenated oils that Joan learned about from her mother, then later from her peers and through her own Internet research).

As the next section will show, women from middle- and upper-class backgrounds—as well as some mixed-class women with high levels of education—were well versed in crafting narratives like Joan's to explain their health and body-care choices. Such narratives put a premium on expertise, both that of health professionals and the expertise women developed through their engagement with health and science knowledge. Ultimately, middle- and upper-class women's narratives about health, reproductive body projects, and taste helped them advance explicit claims about their values and identities. These women did not all share the same values and identities—indeed, one of the hallmarks of these women's stories was how diverse their approaches were—but they all shared a tendency to claim their body projects as empirical evidence of their values. The subsequent section, on poor and working-class mothers, will then explore the limits of self-identity as a concept for understanding the lives and accounts of less privileged subjects.

## Middle-Class Mothers Maintaining Coherent Self-Identities

Women's experiences of becoming pregnant, giving birth, and learning to mother involve change, both physical and mental/emotional. Certainly, many of my respondents noted the ways their bodies and relationships were altered as a result of the transition to parenthood. Yet, among the middle- and upper-class women I spoke to, one of the strongest themes that emerged was constancy: in their habits and practices of caring for themselves, and in their long-standing sense of self-identity and moral commitments. This finding complements the research of Lucy Bailey, who examined first-time pregnancy as an opportunity for changes in self-concept but found, rather, the theme of an augmented—but consistent—identity (terming this phenomenon the "refracted self").[6] In the course of describing how they cared for their bodies during and after pregnancy, several of the middle- and upper-class women I interviewed made reference to their self-care regimens prior to becoming mothers. For these women, most of whom hailed from middle- and upper-class family backgrounds, the notion of a modifiable, trainable body was consistent with the ways they had learned to "do health" prior to having children.

### "I've Just Had Good Eating Habits": Consistency in Middle-Class Food and Diet

Sonia Gallo (Latina, thirty-five, HH) noted that cutting out alcohol was the only significant change she made when she was pregnant. She explained, "[My husband and I] eat pretty healthy. Obviously try to stay away from certain things that you're not supposed to be consuming, [like] alcohol on a rough day. So we don't do that, or if I did, it was a tiny amount, just to wet your tongue. But I wouldn't say we changed our eating too much. . . . We just pretty much ate whatever was normal or whatever we currently eat."

Sonia added that while she made sure to listen to her doctor's advice about alcohol and taking care while exercising during her pregnancies, "the things that were common knowledge are common knowledge." In other words, most of the health practices associated with responsible pregnant embodiment were things she intuitively knew and did already. Charlotte Moran (biracial, thirty-two, HH) told me about her preference for "whole foods" over processed foods (exclaiming, in mock horror, that "processed foods are the devil's work!"). Once Charlotte became pregnant, she became more risk aware but found that she did not need to make many big changes: "I paid a lot more attention to what I was eating. I think I've always eaten well, a balanced diet. . . . I think I've just always had good eating habits." As discussed in chapter 2, pre-parenthood habits formed the foundation for middle- and upper-class women's reproductive body projects, and these women made a point of emphasizing such consistency in the narratives they shared.

Whereas Sonia and Charlotte each drew a straight line from pre-pregnancy health consciousness to their current habits, Lara Noble (white, forty, HH) had a harder time connecting the dots. Lara's mother had written in Lara's baby book decades earlier that "Lara is the most un-liberated little girl. All she talks about is that she wants to be a nurse and a teacher and a mommy." Lara—who had since gone on to work as a professor of nursing—exclaimed, "Look what I am! At age four, that is what I was talking about. Now I teach nursing, and I'm a mommy." In this sense, Lara had a coherent narrative of self-identity that she could trace back to her childhood. Her health history, however, was harder to integrate into that narrative. She recounted, "I had partied pretty substantially in my twenties and thirties. I had sampled everything, but mostly drinking by the time [I wanted to get pregnant]. And I smoked cigarettes, hard-core, for about ten years. . . . And so I knew on a gut level that that was probably adversely affecting things. . . . I had a LEEP procedure and I had pre[cancerous] cervical cells everywhere. They chopped off the end of my cervix. I knew that, from a fertility stand-point, wanting to be a mom, I needed to quit all that." In her late thirties, doctors informed Lara that she had few viable eggs remaining and only a 5 percent chance of conceiving. Whether or not Lara's history of drug and alcohol use directly impacted her fertility, those behaviors were cer-tainly at odds with the social norms of "anticipatory motherhood" that urge all potentially pregnant people to limit their health risks.[7] And so, faced with these dire predictions from her doctors, Lara embarked on a reproductive body project that she believed would boost her chances of conceiving. She added, "I was kind of gearing up. I knew about the folic acid [supplements recommended for early pregnancy]. I knew that there were certain things you needed to do when you became pregnant. I started going to bed a lot earlier. I started eating healthier, probably. I've always been a really healthy eater, despite the drinking and smoking, and I was always a hard-core exerciser."

Despite more than a decade of admittedly less-than-optimal health practices, Lara reframed her story to assert that she had a solid founda-tion of health knowledge and good eating and exercise practices that could help her achieve a successful pregnancy. And, to Lara's mind, those practices made a difference: despite what she was told were long odds, she conceived and carried two pregnancies with ease. She con-cluded, "I feel kind of weird saying it, but I did really feel like I was born to be pregnant." What is striking about Lara's account is the extent to which she glosses over her past unhealthful behaviors in the interest of presenting a consistent narrative about herself as a health-conscious, worthy mother ("I've always been a really healthy eater . . . and I was always a hard-core exerciser").

Consistency was a key theme in the stories of the middle- and upper-class women I interviewed: their eating and exercise habits prior to and during pregnancy differed mainly in terms of degree rather than of kind (adopting a wholly different attitude or approach to the body). Worth noting here is that these mothers may well have selectively edited their accounts of past healthcare habits in order to present a more coherent narrative of themselves and their values; certainly, that was the case for Lara. Such retrospective editing is common in the larger project of self-making, in which both attentive body care *and* coherent self-narratives about that body care play a role.

Key to many of these stories was that, for many middle- and upper-class women, the continuities between their pre- and post-baby self-care practices represented not just a consistent set of habits but a way of being: an identity. As Stephanie Brewer (white, thirty-two, HH) put it, "I've always had a diet that's very low in processed foods, I've always had a diet that's very low in junk. *I've never been an empty calorie person*" (emphasis added). Mixed-class Kirsten Cooper (white, thirty-eight, LH), who had studied nutrition and food science at one of the community colleges she attended, remarked, "I've found that people's food practices are so different than mine! . . . I was never into chips and things like that, but *some people are chip people*" (emphasis added). In their choice of words, both Kirsten and Stephanie described themselves as being particular types of people: avoiding chips or empty calories was not just something they did; it was who they *were*.

### "I've done triathlons, so I can handle this!": Middle-Class Athletic Identities

Although not nearly as widespread as women's comments about diet-based identities, a substantial minority of my middle- to upper-class respondents also emphasized a passionate identification with exercise and athletics. With an average age of 33.7 in the years of my study, middle- and upper-class women I interviewed were mainly born in the mid- to late 1970s. Title IX, part of federal regulations requiring equal opportunities for men and women in education (including interscholastic athletics), was passed in 1972. Thus, most of the mothers in my study came of age at a time when women were increasingly supported in joining competitive sports, pursuing athletic scholarships, and otherwise incorporating athleticism into their personal and professional lives. For many of my subjects, then, managing an "athletic self" became an additional issue to juggle when they became pregnant.

Misty Clifford (white, thirty-one, HH) described the challenges she faced in dealing with the body changes of pregnancy: "I've always been fit. I've always had a pretty healthy body, having been a swimmer. So that was difficult. But when I was showing, it was fun." Misty later told me that she had continued regular jogging into her eighth month of pregnancy; underlying her comments about fitness during pregnancy, then, was a concern not with her activity level but with her slim appearance of *looking* fit (and her anxiety about being perceived as fat). Once she was visibly pregnant—and not merely thicker-waisted than usual—Misty's discomfort with her body lessened.

In a different vein, Suzanne Walsh (white, thirty-five, HH) connected her expectations for pregnancy to her preexisting athleticism: "Because I was such a strong athlete I was like, 'Of course I'm going to have natural childbirth.' My mom had natural childbirth and she's very fit. So there's something about athleticism and natural childbirth that I thought went hand in hand." For Suzanne, her inability to deliver her child without medical intervention felt like an indictment of her athletic, pain-tolerant self. Suzanne took pride in her strength, and she felt such shame at needing medication to help with her delivery that she hesitated to share her birth story with friends. Fiona Garcia expressed a nearly identical sentiment about her eventual Caesarian section, saying, "[Childbirth is] something that I always thought women could get through, and I've done triathlons, so I was like, 'I can handle this.' So, [having the C-section] was a little disappointing."

Although Fiona's and Suzanne's childbirth experiences represented, to them, a failure to maintain a coherent, athletic self-identity while becoming mothers, a key point in these stories is that, once again, exercise was a significant component of their self-concept; their so-called failures were disappointing not because they harmed their children but because they disrupted the women's stable sense of athletic selves.

Middle- and upper-class mothers were not the only ones in my study who placed a high value on athleticism, but it *was* primarily these women who connected their athletic identities to reproductive body projects. For example, LaDonna Douglas (Black, eighteen, LL) was a rising high school senior who hoped to attend college on an athletic scholarship. LaDonna was a serious basketball player who placed a premium on physical fitness, but when I asked her about changes she made to her body-care practices during pregnancy, she responded, "They [health-care providers] said I couldn't run, I couldn't do nothing. I couldn't play sports." I asked LaDonna how she felt about that, and she said, "It just made me out of shape. I felt bad because I know it's going to take me a long time to get back."

Although moderate exercise in pregnancy is recommended by the American College of Obstetricians and Gynecologists (ACOG),[8] out-dated ideas and myths about the risks of exercising while pregnant persist; such myths include worries that raising one's heart rate could deprive the fetus of oxygen or that the jostling motion of running could disrupt the pregnancy. In fact, obstetricians view many types of exercise as beneficial to pregnancy health and warn only against contact sports or those (like downhill skiing or mountain biking) that have a heightened risk for falls. Although competitive high school basketball—LaDonna's preferred form of exercise—can be a full-contact sport, a more person-alized approach might have counseled her to find ways to modify the exercise to help her stay active throughout her pregnancy. From my own observations of WIC offices in California and Florida, I witnessed counselors mentioning "staying active" as important for families, but that was as far as their advice typically went; the vast majority of their advice to pregnant women and parents focused on nutrition. One pam-phlet from a California WIC office—entitled "Give Your Baby a Healthy Start!"—included pregnancy topics such as weight gain, substance use, breastfeeding, and exercise. The pamphlet's only concrete advice about pregnancy exercise suggested, "Talk to your doctor about what is best for you. Walking or other gentle exercise helps you feel good. Think of a safe place, maybe a park or a mall, where you can take walks. Try to walk every day."

While this kind of one-size-fits-all advice may be necessary for a printed pamphlet, it is not clear that low-income women have better luck receiving advice about prenatal exercise from medical providers. As Khiara Bridges details in her ethnography of pregnancy care at an urban hospital, prenatal education about lifestyle risks is often cursory and imperative. She concludes, "It might be more appropriate to regard the program of knowledge given to the patients by [nurses] as *training*."[9] In contrasting education with "training," Bridges emphasizes the disciplinary function of the pregnancy care she observed; health information imparted in this way tends to take the form of directives— prenatal dos and don'ts—rather than responsively meeting patients wherever they are.

Bridges's assessment of prenatal programs targeting low-income women as "training" aligns with my own observations at WIC: counselors and providers working to manage risk and gently—but firmly— bringing clients into compliance with a monolithic biomedical model of health. As a result, there was minimal time left for building on clients' preexisting exercise preferences or limitations. In contrast to upper-middle-class mothers like Misty Clifford, who prioritized working out through their whole pregnancies, or women like Fiona Garcia, who treated their reproductive body projects as an extension of their athletic selves, LaDonna and other athletic low-income mothers more often experienced maternal embodiment as *disruptive to* their athletic identities.

## "That's what I'm programmed to do—I read, I try to solve a problem": Deploying Professional Identities at Home

Finally, one of the biggest challenges to middle- and upper-class women's construction and maintenance of a coherent self during the transition to motherhood was the loss of career-based identities. Sociologists have often noted that motherhood, for women, tends to act as a *master status*, overriding other aspects of self-identity and social status to become the most salient feature of an individual. Describing the condition of women professors, Dorothy Smith explains, "The bifurcation of consciousness becomes for us a daily chasm which is to be crossed, on the one side of which is this special conceptual activity of thought, research, teaching, administration and on the other the world of concrete practical activities in keeping things clean, managing somehow the house and household and the children, a world in which the particularities of persons in their full organic immediacy (cleaning up the vomit, changing the diapers, as well as feeding) are inescapable."[10]

Most of the middle- and upper-class women I interviewed resisted this bifurcation and strove to maintain a coherent professional self-identity, a struggle that was made more difficult by the fact that most women in my study experienced interruptions in their work schedules after having children. Some opted to stay home to care for children full-time, while others scaled back or altered their work commitments, such as through negotiating for more flexibility to work from home or moving into self-employed consulting work. Many observers have speculated about a potential crisis of identity that unemployed men might face during periods of economic recession. However, my interviews suggest that professional women, too, experience serious challenges to identity when they weather even temporary and anticipated interruptions in their careers. These women tried, with varying degrees of success, to translate their work-based personae and skills to meet the requirements of motherhood.

Amy Chen (Asian, thirty-five, HH) described the identity challenges involved in becoming a full-time stay-at-home mother. Following the birth of her first child, Amy returned to work in her corporate job full-time, but changed her plans when her son became critically ill with a virus he caught at daycare. Her husband, a medical school professor, did not consider leaving his job. She explained how drastically she had to readjust her sense of self: "At first I never thought that I could be a stay-at-home mom. . . . The thought never crossed my mind. But I think it was when Alex got sick a *lot*, it kind of made me prioritize things. [But] prior to my son being born I always thought, 'I'm going, I'm working. There's no way I'm not going to work.'" Amy added that this experience was common among the highly educated women in her social circle. Reflecting on the story of one of her friends, she told me, "It's hard to leave something you've worked so hard for. And [my friend] spent $120,000 on law school and developed this career and she left it because of her children. That's something remarkable. To give up something that is a big part of her personality. She's still a pretty Type A personality, and she runs her household like that."

Identifying as "Type A"—that is, as ambitious, competitive, and driven—was common among working women in my study; mothers tried, with varying degrees of success, to apply their "Type A" personalities to their new identities as mothers and their new daily routines centering on what Dorothy Smith calls the "full organic immediacy" of managing children's bodies. Cass Blackwell (white, thirty-three, LH) said, "I have a big perfectionist streak which has served me well in all my jobs and other facets of my life, but it does not serve you well when you become a mother, because you just expect way too much from yourself." And Lee Mendoza (white, thirty, HL) applied her achievement-oriented personality to her mothering when she ran into difficulties breastfeeding: "There was no *rational* reason why I felt so bad about [having trouble breastfeeding], but I think it was my reaction to that burden: 'I have to do this, and no one else can do it. I have to make it work.' And I'm so Type A. I had that goal of [breastfeeding for] one year, and I'm like, 'I will make it to that goal if it kills me!'"

As in Giddens's description of the links between self-identity and lifestyle planning, Lee outlined the connections between her own identity and intentional actions she planned to take: she characterized herself as a particular type of person ("Type A"), and set goals (breastfeeding for a full year) that would bolster that identity. Yet, while Lee's "Type A" tendencies led her to set goals for good mothering habits, she also suspected that part of her difficulties with breastfeeding might have arisen from her stress over meeting a self-imposed benchmark. Thus, both she and Cass expressed serious reservations about the extent to which a "perfectionist," "Type A" personality was compatible with being an effective mother. Perhaps not coincidentally, both Lee and Cass were upwardly mobile, mixed-class women whose outsider status afforded them a more critical perspective on middle-class mothering expectations.

Reconciling professional and parenting identities was a particular challenge for Greta Davies (white, forty, HH). Greta had resigned from her position as a geological researcher to stay at home full-time with her children. Although she did not say that she regretted this choice, she nevertheless struggled to reconcile her identity as a mother with the identity she had established as a scientist: "I find that I'm the one that's doing almost all the parenting, which is hard. I've had a job—I was a geologist—so it's hard to go from working and having colleagues and being a professional to then parenting small children." Greta wondered aloud to me whether her driven, problem-solving professional persona made it harder for her to relax and go with the flow of childrearing, but then she shrugged the conflict off as inevitable: "I don't think you can [avoid building up your expectations], because you read, and that's what I'm programmed to do—I'm a geologist. I read. I try to solve a problem. And I go to my literature, and I go to the Internet, and that's how I deal with life." Although Greta had left her job some time ago, her continued identification as a professional scientist was central to her sense of self and her approaches to parenting. The context in which she deployed her hard-won skills had changed, but their importance to her self-identity remained clear.

Overall, a large number of middle- and upper-class women I spoke to highlighted the ways in which their long-standing identities as con- scientious eaters, tough athletes, and/or trained professionals related to their new, maternal selves. Even at times when embodied experiences of motherhood forced them to adjust their expectations, mothers in my study nevertheless used those preexisting identities to explain some of their feelings about motherhood and to construct consistent narra- tive arcs for themselves. This enduring sense of self voiced by so many middle- and upper-class mothers not only helped them make sense of their past experiences and feelings but also led them to make particular choices about self-care and parenting in the present.

## Middle- and Mixed-Class Women's Negative Comparison Groups: Dissimilar Mothers as Others

While some middle- and upper-class mothers used their reproductive body projects as evidence to positively claim normative identities, many also staked identity claims by contrasting their lifestyles and choices to those of other women. As discussed in chapter 1, middle- and upper- class women counted their peers among their most trusted sources of advice, and many such mothers described choosing their friends on the basis of shared health and parenting values. At the same time, in many mothers' stories there lurked a shadow comparison group: rarely named or explicitly acknowledged, these were particular mothers who formed a negative comparison group against whom middle- and upper-class women could measure themselves.

## *Middle-Class Peers*

Fiona Garcia (white, thirty-nine, HH) differentiated between her own eating habits and those of her husband, explaining, "I'm just not somebody that's into extremes. I've never been the type of person that would sit down and eat a whole bag of potato chips." Likewise, Stephanie Brewer explained her choice to moderate her eating during pregnancy by saying, "I didn't want to be one of those people who started eating a pint of ice cream every day, because . . . I knew it would be really easy to gain sixty pounds and never lose it." Stephanie added that going too far to the other extreme would be problematic, too, describing a pregnant acquaintance who was too "image obsessed": "[She's] having a baby in a few weeks, and she just advertised [on Facebook] yesterday that she went for a mile-long swim, and she went to her doctor afterwards and she'd only gained eighteen pounds. And she's thirty-five weeks!"

For both Stephanie and Fiona, references to others who were, in Fiona's words, "into extremes" became a way to frame their own choices as balanced, moderate, and morally worthy. Perhaps not surprisingly, though, one woman's moderation was another woman's extreme. Stephanie had developed a comprehensive schedule for introducing solid foods to her children, based on her own interpretation of medical guidance for children who were at higher risk of developing food allergies. She typed this schedule into a spreadsheet and shared it, on request, with mothers in her social circle. To mixed-class Lee Mendoza, though, such behavior was "crazy": "[During pregnancy] I was very conscientious about calcium and things for [my daughter's] brain development, probably overly conscientious. I didn't really track it or anything. I'm sure there are people who have spreadsheets, [but] I did not have spreadsheets or anything crazy like that."

In some cases, women overcame cognitive dissonance in order to identify their health habits as moderate and balanced. Greta Davies, for example, told me about her insistence on limiting her children's sugar intake. She took away their Halloween candy and, in response to a bank teller who asked to give her daughter a lollipop, she exclaimed, "Why would you ask me that? No you can't!" Yet, describing her recent interaction with another mother, Greta went to great pains to paint herself as "not obsessive": "You start off by giving kids Cheerios for a little snack, and one woman was like 'Oh, Trader O's [the store-brand version of Cheerios sold at Trader Joe's grocery stores] are better.' I'm like, 'What's wrong with Cheerios?' 'Too much sugar.' I'm like, 'Are you kidding me? It's Cheerios!' And that's the level of obsessiveness . . . that people are at today. And I'm like, 'That's insane!'"

Mothers' comparisons to similarly situated peers with different values often hinged on judgments about which health and parenting behaviors they perceived to be balanced, moderate, and sensible, and which were "crazy," "insane," or "extreme." In accordance with late modern self-identity formation's dependence on self-reflection, these women had considered their own approaches carefully and developed a narrative for why they made those particular choices (as well as what differing choices said about other parents). This practice enabled them to assert not only particular types of values but also claims to being a particular type of self: an enduring sense of identity tied to their status as mothers and their membership in a privileged class.

To be clear, none of the middle- and upper-class mothers I interviewed spoke too disparagingly about the choices of mothers they knew personally (with the exception, perhaps, of their own mothers). Far from the passive-aggressive jockeying that media depictions of the so-called Mommy Wars highlight, I suggest that most women in this group discursively othered their peers for one of two reasons. First, the imperative to make ongoing, dedicated body projects a central part of their self-identity as women and mothers required my subjects to define clearly their own health values; the simplest way to do so was by comparison to others. Second, few of these women viewed themselves as crusaders for health; more often, they explained their choices defensively, as if anticipating judgment from others. Thus, their comments may represent a half-conscious acknowledgment of the disciplining pressures exerted by other women's health practices and by healthist norms in society more generally. If peers from a mother's reference group pursue increasingly demanding health and body projects, she has two options: to follow along, or to narratively frame her eschewal of those practices as a reasoned choice in line with her personal health goals (thereby reaffirming the normative value of prioritizing health even as she rejects particular practices as being peripheral to that pursuit). In line with the risk-assessing paradigm discussed in the previous chapter, women who engaged in health and body-care practices that fell short of the "extremes" of the risk-avoidant approach believed that they needed to discursively frame their choices as scientific and well-researched or face the scorn of their peers. In essence, by anticipating judgment from their peers, mothers internalized disciplinary norms for body care; by outspokenly defending their choices and enumerating all they did to optimize their children's bodies and well-being, they contributed to the very climate they feared.

### Upper- and Mixed-Class Mothers, Working-Class Others

On rarer occasions, HH and mixed-class mothers used poor and working-class women as their negative reference group. Nadia Bernard (white, thirty-six, HH) was one of the few to name low-income mothers explicitly. She recounted, "I was online watching some show. And they have the macaroni and cheese in a bag now. So you just open the bag, dump it in a [pan], and bake it in the oven. I was just like, yuck! [making a face] I have my limits. You know, the food is now the thing that separates [classes]. . . . It's a marker of class more than cars, more than clothes, more than anything else." For Nadia, even knowing that access to healthy food was tied to class privilege did not prevent her from asserting (by making a disgusted face and stating, "I have my limits") that her food choices were morally righteous.

In other cases, mothers drew distinctions on the basis of disparities in information and health literacy. Most highly educated women I interviewed believed that taking proper care of oneself and one's children required extensive knowledge and expertise. Mixed-class Christine Webber (white, thirty-seven, HL) said of her special diet for gestational diabetes, "You have to have a degree in rocket science to figure it out." Christine did not have a degree in rocket science, but she did have two graduate degrees. Stephanie Brewer, who was frustrated with the contradictory advice often given to pregnant and breastfeeding mothers, added, "[It] creates a lot of confusion among very educated mothers. Imagine what kind of confusion it's creating for mothers who maybe don't have enough education to be able to analyze what's there and make a decision." Stephanie and Christine both spoke sympathetically about how difficult it would be to make good choices without their high levels of education, but implicit in their statements was the notion that women with less education probably made worse health choices.

Mixed-class Frankie Ford (white, twenty-six, LH) was more explicitly judgmental. Frankie managed a gas station and observed the spending habits of lower-income women, saying, "I've never gotten food stamps, but we do food stamps here [at the gas station convenience store], and I see people get twelve-packs of soda. I've seen them get thirty dollars of candy and Red Bull. I don't know how that qualifies as feeding your family with money that's supposed to be helping you feed your family healthy. . . . I disapprove of how they do it." Frankie believed that WIC was superior to food stamps because it did more to limit participants' choices to foods Frankie perceived to be healthy. Describing a recent policy change at WIC (in which adults and older children could no longer receive vouchers for full-fat milk), Frankie drew a contrast between her own outlook and that of most WIC recipients: "I was the only person—there were probably about six other [clients] in the room—I was the only one that wasn't totally throwing a fit about [the change to low-fat milk]. I was just like, 'This is supposed to make you healthy. I don't understand why you guys are going nuts about it, if they're trying to help you.'"

Frankie framed her fellow WIC recipients as unreasonable, unhealthy, and—in the case of those who also received SNAP/food stamp benefits—wasteful, thereby identifying herself as health conscious and thrifty in comparison. For mixed-class women like Frankie, who stood with one foot in the middle class and one foot in the working class, their class position made them both aware of middle-class habits and criteria for "good motherhood" and also self-conscious about being associated with poorer women. They engaged in a variety of cross-class boundary-drawing practices to establish their identities and distinguish themselves from low-income mothers.

Solidly middle- and upper-class women were less likely to feel at risk of being lumped in with low-income mothers, and so their references to such women were minimal. Instead, their negative reference groups were predominantly same-class peers: women with whom they regularly interacted in larger peer circles and "mommy groups," but whose choices they deemed "obsessive" or "extreme" in order to frame their own practices as sensible and moderate. As their contrast with mixed-class women demonstrates, middle- and upper-class women's ability to use same-status peers as their negative reference groups for self-identity is itself a marker of privilege; there was little chance of their being mistaken for the kind of "bad" low-income mother who, in Gita Potter's words, was "the kind of person who eats macaroni and cheese for every meal." These mothers, if they took notice of low-income women at all, tended to express sympathy for mothers who lacked the education to understand a complex diet or the money to buy organic produce. Yet, by maintaining that such practices were ideal for self- and child care, they were asserting—however softly—that their mothering practices and identities were superior to those of most poor and working-class women. Thus, regardless of the material consequences of these practices (that is, whether they actually produce better outcomes later in life), the middle- and upper-class mothers I spoke to implicitly linked their practices to class advantage and status transmission.

## Low-Income Women and Disidentification

Middle- and upper-class women's reproductive body projects made ready resources for staking self-identity claims in the stories they told about themselves. But these ties between identity and body projects did not arise uniformly across demographics: as this next section will show, poor and working-class mothers were often hesitant to make their reproductive body projects the basis for identity claims. Instead, when recounting their decisions about nutrition, exercise, consumption of medical care, and more, these women explained those choices as a result of personal weakness or failure or, in other cases, as an expression of personal taste that did not rise to the level of an identity.

### "They said it's better for the baby": Personal Failure Frames

Poor and working-class mothers frequently measured themselves against the monolithic health standards promoted by WIC. Faced with a single standard for "good" health practices—but having limited resources for attaining it—many low-income women admitted that they thought their own health practices fell short. Lynne O'Brien (white, twenty-seven, LL) explained her decision to stop breastfeeding her youngest child thus:

"I did cheat because I was going back and forth from breastfeeding to bottle feeding. I think [switching over to formula feeding] was more or less my laziness at that point because I do have so many kids, and it is harder to deal with at that point than it was [with previous children]." Throughout her interview, Lynne noted specific circumstances that made it hard to breastfeed: physical exhaustion, pain, and the complicated logistics of breastfeeding an infant while simultaneously caring for two other young children. Nevertheless, the language she used to describe her choice framed it as a personal failure to achieve something she considered ideal. Introducing a bottle was "cheating," and succumbing to exhaustion was "laziness."

A number of low-income women used similar frames of personal responsibility, explaining their "bad" choices as the result of personal deficits and preferences. Sarah Evans (white, twenty-one, LL), currently pregnant with her second child, had suffered through gestational diabetes and other health problems during her first pregnancy. She recalled family friends telling her that she should watch her diet and get more exercise, but said she responded by saying, "'Yeah, whatever.' I just wouldn't listen to them. Because when someone says something more than once and they just keep pushing it, it just gets on your nerves. . . . It would have helped, though, if I had listened instead of being so hardheaded." Sarah, like many women, was uncomfortable with the public nature of her pregnant body. Facing constant bodily scrutiny "gets on your nerves," and Sarah resisted this normalizing judgment by doing her best to ignore it. Retrospectively, however, she viewed her weight gain and ill health as the product of her stubbornness ("being so hardheaded") and now, in her second pregnancy, she aimed to do better. When Sarah had her first child, she was hospitalized for pneumonia and ended up having to give her son formula. She regretted not breastfeeding, saying, "They said it's better for the baby. And I always wanted to do it because they say it builds [babies'] immune system up. I wish I would have did it, because ever since he's been born [it's been] one thing and another with sickness, like ear infections."

Sarah's description of the breastfeeding ideal—"they said it's better for the baby"—framed it both as good and as being externally imposed, rather than as a practice she innately felt to be best. Indeed, Sarah had lingering doubts about what "they said" about the benefits of breastfeeding: her little brother was exclusively breastfed yet dealt with a lot of health problems, so, she mused, "I don't really know how true it is [that breastfeeding prevents illness]." Still, she was determined to try harder with her next child.

### "I want to set a good example, but I don't like it": Personal Taste Frames

Whereas Sarah and Lynne ascribed the gap between their body-care practices and the norm to personal *failures*, many more low-income women emphasized the role of personal *tastes*. In some cases, mothers' tastes led them to reject WIC-endorsed body-care practices; in other cases, they followed mainstream health norms but did so reluctantly or for a limited period of time. Shontel Sykes (Black, twenty, LL) noted that she did not particularly like the foods WIC recommended but followed their guidelines anyway: "They give you wheat bread. I want to buy white bread. They give you juices. I want to buy soda. If they didn't give me those things I probably wouldn't buy it. It wouldn't be on my mind. [If I wasn't in WIC] I'd probably buy junk food, like chicken, macaroni, fries, burgers. . . . I like things like that, but I try also to get [my son] nutritious things, but it's hard because I don't really eat it myself. I want to set a good example, but it's kind of hard. I don't like it either."

Here, Shontel set up a contrast between how she preferred to eat and the choices she made on behalf of her child. While Shontel's grudging compliance with WIC's advice signals that she accepted WIC's health knowledge as authoritative—she trusted that the eating habits they recommended would benefit her child—she nevertheless wanted to assert that she was a person with her own tastes and preferences. Yet she was also a person who consciously chose to set aside those preferences for the sake of her children.

Many other women also tried to follow dietary advice while simultaneously distancing themselves from it. LaDonna Douglas (Black, eighteen, LL) labeled herself a "picky eater" who struggled to eat the foods WIC recommended: "They do give me fruits and stuff, which I haven't been eating. I really don't eat fruits. . . . I'm like, let me try some new things. I tried grapes and strawberries, cantaloupes. I really don't like them."

During pregnancy, LaDonna did her best to follow the list of food recommendations her doctor had given her, but she still craved foods like pizza and spicy Chinese cuisine that she perceived to be "bad" for pregnancy. Shawna Blanchard (Black, twenty, LL) and Gaby Romero (Latina, twenty-nine, LL) also used the word "picky" to describe themselves relative to mainstream dietary recommendations. Shawna, pregnant with her first child, laughed as she admitted, "Maybe [I should] just stay away from a lot of stuff with sugars. I eat a lot of not-good stuff that I'm [not] supposed to." And Gaby, who was still nursing her first-born, added, "I don't really like to eat a lot of fruit and stuff, but since I been in the program because of the baby, I've been changing my habits of eating. And that, I think, is a good benefit for me and for the baby."

For these women—as for many other low-income women I interviewed—eating the "right way" was only a sporadic part of their reproductive body projects. On one hand, they mostly endorsed WIC-supported dietary norms as healthful, contrasting "good" fruit, vegetables, and whole grains with the "bad" sugary, fatty, salty, spicy foods they desired. On the other hand, they did not identify as the sort of people who enjoyed or sought out the "good" foods. Instead, they identified as "picky" eaters for whom healthy eating did not come naturally. Embedded in that identification, also, was the claim that for these women, eating in normatively healthy ways demonstrated their hard work and willingness to sacrifice for their children.

Similar patterns emerged in respondents' discussions of breastfeeding. WIC, known for many years as the "formula program" because of its provision of free infant formula, had begun working to promote breastfeeding over formula. Most women enrolled in WIC had gotten the message that "breast is best," yet many still did not initiate breastfeeding or stopped after only a couple of days, weeks, or months. For some mothers, logistical concerns like low milk production or inflexible work schedules were barriers to achieving these benchmarks; for others, personal taste and comfort played a role in their decision to add in formula.

Kiara Jefferson (Black, twenty, LL) had mixed feelings about breastfeeding. After her daughter was born, she said, "I put her up to my breast for one time, but I didn't like it." I asked Kiara what about it she didn't like; she explained that "the funny thing about it was the baby's mouth to the nipple. That's why I didn't like it. . . . It was hurting, or just uncomfortable." Kiara was uneasy about the act of breastfeeding but, having absorbed WIC's lessons about the benefits of breastmilk, decided to hand-express milk instead: "All I did was squeeze it in a bottle." I asked whether Kiara used a pump, and she responded, "Nah, I just squeezed it." Throughout her daughter's infancy, Kiara alternated between bottles of hand-expressed milk and formula, but she never offered her breast again.

Meanwhile, Vanessa Garfield (white, twenty-five, LL) felt proud—not guilty—about the relatively short period of time she breastfed her children. She recounted,

> I thought breastfeeding was good for him, and it relieved a lot of the pressure that I had. But it felt like I wasn't producing enough, and I was pumping all day for just a little bit of milk. Pretty much my entire day was pumping, pumping, pumping. It wasn't even enough to make a whole bottle. . . . Even with my second, I still didn't produce enough milk to do it. . . . I did it for two weeks with him. Even if he only got two weeks, I thought it was good for the breastmilk to be in his system. So I did it for as long as I could.

Vanessa's perception that she was not producing enough milk for her child may or may not have been accurate: many new mothers feel unsure about how much milk an infant needs, or how much they are producing (especially if a baby is nursing directly from the breast). In contrast, preparing a bottle of formula is relatively quick and offers visual confirmation that the baby is getting fed. Vanessa, like Kiara and many other women I spoke to, reconceptualized the role of breastfeeding in her overall reproductive body project: she did not reject the dominant medical opinion that breastmilk was the healthiest food to give babies, but neither did she identify herself as a bad mother for failing to breastfeed in the "right way" (exclusive of formula, for six months or longer). Instead, like low-income mothers who described themselves as "picky eaters," Vanessa and others incorporated medically normative practices into their reproductive body projects in ways that were partial or temporary. In so doing, poor and working-class mothers highlighted the work that these projects required: they did not identify as the sort of people for whom such changes were natural or inevitable, but rather as people whose preferences ran counter to the dominant health norm (and who were sacrificing their own comfort to do what they had been told was best for their children).

## Self-Identity and Disidentification

In the examples described above, poor and working-class women state that they accept at least some parts of dominant health ideologies (regarding diet, the superiority of breastmilk, and more), but they simultaneously distance themselves from those ideologies. Citing personal tastes or weaknesses, they emphasize not the *closeness* between what they believe is best and how they act but the *distance*. This does not line up with Giddens's notion of lifestyle-based self-identity cultivation, and it is a far cry from the narratives that middle- and upper-class women told me (about how their preexisting identities as athletes or professional researchers informed their transition to motherhood). How, then, should we understand poor and working-class women's accounts?

José Esteban Muñoz introduces the term "disidentification" for understanding how some minoritized people respond to dominant social norms and identities that exclude them. Writes Muñoz, disidentification is an approach that "neither opts to assimilate within [dominant ideology] nor strictly opposes it; rather, disidentification is a strategy that works on and against dominant ideology."[11] In the case of poor and working-class mothers, disidentification is a possible defense against a system that offers only two identities: the "good" mother who gladly complies with all health directives and provides for all of her children's needs, or the "bad" mother who fails to do so. When mothers emphasize how difficult and distasteful WIC-recommended dietary guidelines are, they are not directly contesting the health benefits of, say, eating fruits and vegetables. Instead, they are carving out a space for themselves: if not as the "right" kinds of subjects who eat greens and like them, then at least as mothers who care enough about their children to do something they dislike.

Furthermore, whereas middle- and upper-class mothers seemed comfortable using their health and body-care practices to stake identity claims, poor and working-class mothers frequently resisted making those connections: disidentification, for them, was not about crafting identities but about resisting the expectation that their practices should become the basis for an identity at all. This is not to say that poor and working-class women had no identities, or no desire to represent themselves in a positive light. But they often responded negatively to the expectation that they define themselves through their embodied consumption practices or through the lens of healthism. Middle- and upper-class mothers' cultural and economic resources allowed them to personalize their reproductive body projects to reflect their tastes and preferences and integrate them into their sense of self. Private health insurance plans and an ability to pay out of pocket when insurance did not cover these preferences allowed women to choose a healthcare provider who endorsed their pursuit of particular health goals (rather than going with whichever provider accepted Medicaid), and to find some external validation for scientifically unsupported practices. Expansive grocery budgets enabled women to choose organic, low-carb, or other specialized foods, rather than the limited selection of "healthful" foods covered by WIC. And for those with the means to pay, specialists like personal trainers, dietitians, and doulas can partner with women to deliver personalized body projects that reflect clients' individual needs and values.

In contrast, poor and working-class mothers had fewer options for expressing themselves through consumption choices because their choices were financially limited. WIC, for example, subsidizes low-income families' food budgets through vouchers for foods it deems nutritious, but does not cover the spices and cooking oils that would make such foods palatable; instead of offering personalized nutrition plans, WIC counselors are authorized only to facilitate clients' compliance with a single standard for healthful eating. Diya, a WIC nutritionist in Florida, showed me her computer screen and described the bureaucratic work of assembling a client's monthly food voucher allowances thus:

We created a cheat sheet in here for commonly prescribed food packages. These are the ones for those low-risk [clients] that don't take very much time: children one to two; infant core packages. These are the different formulas; this is how much they get. For women, if they want cheese or no cheese, beans, and peanut butter. [For] breastfeeding and partially breastfeeding women. . . . Before, as a prenatal [client], we only had the option of beans or peanut butter. Now we have the option of beans and peanut butter. You get a little less of each, but you get both in the same month.

In the WIC office, "personalization" looked like a client's ability to swap out eggs or cheese for another protein-rich item if they had an allergy, or the ability to access both beans and peanut butter in a single month. Within the computerized systems for managing benefits, even authorizing an alternative infant formula—one not covered by the state's exclusive contract with a formula manufacturer—required a doctor's note and time-consuming work-arounds. Alternative formulas were available only to babies with a demonstrated medical need (for example, a soy-based formula for a baby with dairy allergies), rather than on the basis of the baby's or parent's tastes. Certainly, WIC made few allowances for dietary preferences like the vegetarian, low-carb, or "primal"/paleo diets that were common among higher-class women.

Given both WIC's inflexibility and low-income mothers' lack of disposable income for pursuing personalized body projects, the health-related practices these women described to me were compromises: the result of their efforts to do their best with limited resources. Rather than serving as a pure reflection of their values, these women's consumption choices reflect their efforts to make do with what was available. These compromises born of necessity, along with women's self-effacing comments about "laziness" or "pickiness," indicate that low-income mothers did not see their body-care practices as a special source of pride or self-identity.

Lastly, the types of disidentificatory responses women described hint at racialized class patterns of disidentification: poor and working-class white women were more likely to label themselves and their reproductive body projects with negative descriptors ("lazy," "hard-headed," etc.) and also more likely to admit to cigarette and/or drug use (five out of ten working-class white women recounted cigarette use, while none of the poor/working-class women of color reported it). In contrast, low-income women of color were somewhat more likely to highlight taste-based disidentifications (e.g., "I try to follow health guidelines but I don't like it"). These differences may reflect the fact that while all mothers are subject to normative judgment, racist assumptions in society make women of color more vulnerable to being labeled "bad mothers." In response, these women—Black and Latina mothers in particular—may have been more careful not only in making health decisions (being, both in the current project and in nationally representative studies, less likely to smoke cigarettes) but also in choosing how to frame information they disclosed about themselves. Both the "personal failure" and "personal taste" forms of disidentification, however, were similar in that they emphasized low-income mothers' distance from consumer-based health practices rather than positively articulating these women's identities and values.

## Alternative Identifications among Poor, Working-Class, and Mixed-Class Women

There were a few notable exceptions to the patterns of disidentification described above: upwardly mobile women, devoutly religious women, and first- or second-generation immigrants often wove narratives of alternative identities and values. Such identities were based in these women's strong cultural ties to a community that afforded them a viable alternative to mainstream health-focused identities.

### Alternative Immigrant Identities: Asian and Latina Mothers

Immigrant mothers, who had ties to other cultures, were among those most likely to call out US mainstream health norms as culturally specific. Mexican immigrant Luz Flores (Latina, twenty-eight, LL) described her difficulty getting health and diet advice from her best friend due to their different cultural backgrounds: "My friend is different, everybody in this country is different, comes from different countries and have different menus. . . . My friend is from El Salvador, and she is married [to a] Black man. She eats so different than me. And my ex-husband is from Guam, and he's different. This is not something I can talk to her about, because it's a hundred percent different, their routine and everything."

Luz thought a lot about how to make healthful choices for herself and her children, but she also recognized that, across different nations and cultures, there was no universal standard for what such choices might

THE STORIES MOTHERS TELL | 151

look like. Ji-Eun Park (Asian, thirty-five, HL) likewise discussed cultur-ally specific health practices in her interview with me. Ji-Eun had moved with her husband from South Korea to Florida, where he attended grad-uate school. The couple belonged to a local church whose congregation included several nurses and doctors with whom Ji-Eun felt comfortable discussing medical issues. Nevertheless, when Ji-Eun's children were born, she called her parents back home for advice:

> For the treatment of postpartum [bodies], we Koreans have our own method. So I ask my parents and they told me how to take care of my body. For example, after the delivery, we don't go outside for three weeks. And for nutrition, we have special soups for three months. . . . That is a kind of seaweed soup, and it helps for the lactation and also it helps the recovery of the body. And after the three-week period, the Koreans are very careful for everything, not to use the muscles to twist, or don't move too many things. For this, my parents told me many things about prohibitions.

Ji-Eun was not a complete traditionalist; she noted that traditional Korean postpartum care had developed in a context where many people lived in poverty with insufficient nutrition. Living in the contempo-rary United States, she explained, required her to "distinguish which [approach] is right for me here and now." She added, "For the three weeks of the special postpartum [care], my parents are definitely right. After that, I need to consider about the scientific field, because my body condition is not exactly the same as the old-style Korean women. I think that I need to know both sides and then I can take what I need."

For immigrant women like Ji-Eun and Luz, exposure to non-US health values and practices provided a critical perspective on the kinds of health norms and advice they faced in the United States. While they often did prioritize the advice they received from WIC staff and other US health professionals, they were aware that "health" was not an objec-tive, universal status but rather, a culturally defined norm. As Ji-Eun pointed out, this perspective allowed her to "know both sides and . . . take what I need." When these women's practices diverged from what WIC and other US health professionals advised, they did not disidentify with mainstream health norms. Instead, they attributed these differences to alternative cultural identifications. In other words, instead of describing their practices as a failure to attain a mainstream healthy identity, they framed those practices as part of rich, alternative ethnic/immigrant identities.

### Alternative Religious Identities: Mixed-Class Mothers

Another group of women who adopted alternative frameworks for health and self-identity were those with strong religious affiliations, almost all of whom were mixed-class. In some cases, religious precepts underlay mothers' reproductive body projects. Such was the case for Gita Potter (Asian, twenty-seven, HL): "I'm LDS [Mormon], so I belong to the Church of Jesus Christ of the Latter-Day Saints, and there's a lot of doctrinal principles, especially about the things we put into our bodies, and not [using] harmful substances like drugs, alcohol, tobacco, things like that."

Many of Gita's religiously imposed health and diet restrictions aligned with mainstream health norms. When I asked her about changes she made during pregnancy, she laughed and noted that she already did not drink alcohol or caffeine, so there was little she needed to change. In this way, Gita's faith bolstered her ability to enact a normative reproductive body project. Noura Berry (white, twenty-three, HL), on the other hand, followed religious traditions that were at odds with mainstream health recommendations. Noura, a Hare Krishna, had spent most of her childhood in India. On the basis of her interpretation of her religion's teachings, Noura followed a strict vegetarian diet and resisted vaccinating her nearly two-year-old son (who, at the time of our interview, was recovering from whooping cough). Noura believed that physical health was closely connected to spiritual and emotional well-being, but she also opposed the notion that illness is something to be avoided at all costs. For example, she confided in me that she hoped her son would contract chicken pox as a child, explaining how she believed this would teach him to tolerate illness: "They can learn about what it means to be sick and how it's okay to stay home and you get some extra time with your mom. I think we've lost it a lot with the vaccination against chicken pox. I mean, why do we do that anyway? Why do we have vaccinations against the flu? Why would we want to be completely healthy all the time, and then suddenly get some chronic illness like cancer and be completely unprepared?"

Noura spoke passionately about her deeply held religious values, her opinions on the body, and the connections she saw between the two. She was untroubled by doctors' negative opinions about how she cared for her own health and her son's; instead, she felt satisfied that by raising her son in accordance with her faith traditions, she was engaging in an ideal reproductive body project. Noura told me she felt guilty about conceiving a child outside of marriage, which violated the tenets of her religious faith. In her mind, raising her son with a vegetarian diet and rejecting vaccines on his behalf were ways for her to reclaim an identity as both a good Hare Krishna and a good mother.[12]

While, for mothers like Noura and Gita, religion provided principles for health and body care (allowing them to access a different sort of healthy identity), in other cases religion served as an *alternative* to health and body-based identification. Annie Castro (white, twenty-nine, HL) described how her Christian identity helped her stop focusing so much on her body: "I struggled with anorexia. And I'd say that it really cleared up when I was nineteen, in college." I asked her what had changed in her relationship to her body, and she said, "I went to a faith-based college and I think that . . . getting my life in order [in terms] of what I believed changed a lot of that. I went more from self-focused to how God sees me."

Annie had spent her teenage years drastically limiting her food intake in pursuit of a slender physique, believing what she later called a "lie that a man told me" that equated her self-worth with her physical appearance. She reflected that her earlier efforts at controlling her body were about seeking outside approval, whether from boyfriends or from society at large. Since her religious awakening, however, Annie described her new orientation toward her body as "content" and "coming to terms" with her body's natural shape, even as she still "want[ed] to take care of it." In making this change, she was trying to relearn how to see her body as "God sees me," not as social norms did. Through her faith tradition, Annie was learning to define her worth and identity beyond her body.

Nicki Lindsay (white, thirty, HL) likewise made religious faith a centerpiece of her sense of identity and self-care. Nicki spent her free time volunteering with her church at a local crisis pregnancy center (one of a network of conservative Christian nonprofit organizations that oppose abortion and offer peer counseling for pregnant women). She had met her husband, a pastor, in college when they attended the same church, and most of her close friends were also members of her church. I asked Nicki what sort of things she did to take care of herself, a question that most middle-class women answered with descriptions of their fitness routines or dietary choices. Nicki, however, responded,

> I do take time for myself. Right now it's two to three p.m., and that is quiet time. . . . It's time for me to do things that I like to do. And right now I've been either reading or praying, and having time to relax. . . . I know a lot of people say that they meditate or do those things for recharging. But praying, for me, definitely recharges me through the power of God to be able to not blow up at the kids later on. . . . I try not to do things like laundry or housework during that time, so that I can be the best mom that I can be.

Nicki added that managing her stress was a particularly important priority, and that "if I have to stand on a treadmill, that would make me more stressed out than anything." For Nicki, exercise felt like one more chore to accomplish, rather than a tool to manage her stress; she preferred quiet prayer as the best way to care for her own needs. Both Nicki and Annie noted the pressures they felt to devote time to working on their bodies. Both acknowledged that *caring* for their bodies remained an important value, but—bolstered by their religious identities—they differentiated between listening to what kind of holistic care their bodies actually needed and simply following normative guidelines for diet and fitness. Annie described her Christian faith as offering her an alternative to a femininity defined by unrealistic beauty norms. And Nicki's assertion that prayer helped her "be the best mom that I can be" set aside appearance-centered feminine identity norms in favor of a more traditional feminine identity grounded in motherhood.

The alternative identifications available to low-income women followed particular demographic patterns. Immigrant women—generally Latina or Asian—tended to find alternative sources of identity and health values in their cultures of origin; alternative identifications based in religion were most common among mixed-class women, especially (but not exclusively) white women living in Florida. The latter were often college educated even as their low household incomes made them eligible for WIC. These women resisted becoming typical WIC clients: as detailed in chapter 1, they often aligned themselves with WIC staff members and distanced themselves from fellow aid recipients. At the same time, participation in the consumption-based identity practices of middle-class women was often financially out of reach for them. Under these circumstances, seeking out community and alternative identity through religious affiliation may have felt particularly meaningful, a way to engage in the self-identity construction process that Giddens claims is demanded by late modernity without having to do so through consumption. Religious identification was particularly salient in northern Florida, which has some of the country's highest levels of residents who self-identify as "very religious," and where "What church do you attend?" is a common conversation starter.

### Alternative Aspirational Identities: Poor and Working-Class Black Women

In contrast to immigrant and mixed-class women, poor and working-class US-born Black women were less likely to cite alternative cultural identities when I asked them about their health and body-care values; these women were among the most likely to disidentify with WIC-approved health norms, making partial changes to their diets or activity for their children's sake while proclaiming their dislike for these changes.

Similar to religious women, however, a handful of low-income Black women found a source of alternative identification through their aspirations toward upward mobility. These women usually did not challenge mainstream health norms but instead voiced alternative values that guided their childrearing and health practices. Nicole Johnson (Black, twenty-two, LL) exemplified this alternative identification. Nicole explained that motherhood made her realize how much care for herself and care for others were connected: "I think, having a kid, you really have to step up everything. In taking care of myself, I have to *really* take care of myself. Even though I have a lot of people depending on me—my little brother and my sister—I have to take care of myself, or what's going to happen to them?"

When Nicole got pregnant at the age of sixteen, she had already been financially supporting her younger siblings for a few years and had been in and out of foster care, due to her mother's drug use and her father's absence. Despite intense morning sickness—which Nicole wryly referred to as "all-the-time sickness"—that caused her to lose more than thirty pounds, Nicole concealed her pregnancy and kept working at a local restaurant chain. On the day she gave birth to her daughter Keshia, Nicole enrolled in WIC. There, staff members urged her to take care of her daughter through health-focused practices: first exclusive breastfeeding, then later various dietary practices. Nicole was enthusiastic about breastfeeding, saying, "I always knew I would breastfeed," and even when women relatives told her it was not worth the pain and difficulty, she responded, "I'm a tough person, so you can't tell me something like that. You can't tell me that I can't just because you can't do it." Nicole managed to nurse Keshia for the better part of eight months. WIC staff urged her to continue to the twelve-month mark, but, Nicole explained, "I was working all different hours, so it was hard and I wasn't pumping enough milk. They weren't understanding that it's not enough for Keshia and then I would have to leave work early. I had to change over [to formula]; it just wasn't working out."

In some ways, Nicole's response to WIC's normative guidance about breastfeeding sounds like disidentification: she acknowledged the good of the ideal they were pushing, but also did not agonize over her failure to meet that ideal when circumstances changed. At the same time, throughout our interview together it became clear that Nicole was driven by a strong sense of purpose. A self-described "tough person," Nicole had worked for pay since she was thirteen years old, doing housekeeping for her middle school vice principal to supplement her family's income. She explained, "I'm the one [in my family] that will take care of everybody. I'm the one that's going to have to go to school, I'm the one that always got to set the example." Nicole had left school when she was in her midteens to work full-time to care for her younger siblings, but when she got pregnant with Keshia she enrolled in an alternative high school for at-risk teens, got her GED, and, when I met her, was working toward a bachelor's degree in education, working part-time, volunteering at a local middle school, and planning on a career as a special education preschool teacher.

I offer Nicole's story to demonstrate how strong a sense of purpose she infused into her narrative of self-identity, but also to note how little that identity was defined by her body-care practices. Nicole, the child of a single, drug-addicted mother and a teen mom and high school dropout herself, was fervently devoted to upward mobility and financial security for herself and her family. When Nicole ceased breastfeeding Keshia, she did so due to her belief that she could best care for her family as a breadwinner. At that point, the uncertain benefits of continuing breastfeeding were outweighed by holding down a job and securing her family's financial future.

While not all respondents painted their stories in such vivid strokes, Nicole's account taps into a Black cultural ideal that underpinned many mothers' stories. As Dawn Dow explains, Black women in the United States struggle less to reconcile their identities as workers with their identities as mothers than white women typically do. Instead, she finds, they adopt an ideology of "integrated mothering" that assumes "mothers will work outside the home, be economically self-reliant, and have access to kin and community members to assist them with child care. These mothers [do] not feel compelled to justify their decisions in order for them to be socially palatable to others."[13] Dow's research suggests that these women's identities as providers enriched, rather than undercut, their identities as caregivers. Likewise, Omise'eke Natasha Tinsley describes how, for many women throughout the African diaspora, labor is a central component of their identities as women and mothers.[14] Nicole and a handful of other working-class Black women frequently answered my questions about how they cared for their families with detailed narratives about financial provision, not dietary regimens, and they expressed no guilt about making pragmatic health and body-care choices that did not fully align with WIC recommendations if they felt that those choices enabled them to meet their family's needs in other ways.

## Conclusion

Across classes, mothers responded in varying ways to the normative demand that they actively construct self-identities through carefully selected "body regimes."[15] Middle- and upper-class mothers tended to embrace this expectation, using diet, exercise, and professional careers to claim identities as particular "types" of people. Most treated pregnancy and other stages of maternal embodiment as opportunities to further develop those identities, rather than as disruptions to identity. They engaged in informed consumption of health products and expert advice, facilitated by both financial resources and cultural capital, and they defined themselves primarily against other middle- and upper-class peers, specifically against mothers whose values were fairly similar to their own. In so doing, they were able to make fine-grained distinctions about the degree of intensity or devotion with which they pursued their reproductive body projects.

Poor and working-class mothers, in contrast, seemed uneasy about the expectation that their health and body-care practices should define their values and identities. Many women in this group engaged in processes of *disidentification*, adopting elements of mainstream medical advice for health—often in partial or temporary ways—while refusing to claim that such practices were easy or natural for them. They did so in the context of participation in WIC, a federal food assistance program whose mission is to instill normative health habits in low-income families and communities. While some women in this group resisted the pressure to internalize these values by disidentifying (often emphasizing that WIC-approved practices were difficult or ran counter to their tastes), others found stability in alternative identities and values: minority ethnic/immigrant identities, religious identities, and identities that redefined care as financial provision rather than consumption.

Mixed-class women tended to fall somewhere in between these two positions. Especially among those who were highly educated yet low-income (HL), mixed-class mothers responded to the demand for health-focused self-identities by distinguishing their health practices and knowledge from those of poorer or less educated women. They lacked the financial resources to enjoy all the trappings of middle- and upper-class reproductive body projects, but took pains to explain that they *knew* about those products and practices and used them whenever they could. A number of these women also pursued alternative identities and body-care priorities through their participation in religious communities. Mixed-class women gave the most explicit statements about the links between body projects and class, likely because of their exposure to both higher- and lower-class women and their anxieties about being

misidentified as poor mothers with "bad" values. These women's narratives, then, functioned as evidence of their allegiance to higher-class
identities and cultural values and distinguished them from economically
similar low-income peers.

What accounts for these class differences in identifications and disidentifications? One piece of the puzzle is that women from different
class backgrounds did, indeed, have different tastes and preferences
that affected the contents of their reproductive body projects. As Pierre
Bourdieu reminds us, class conditions people with limited financial resources to develop a "taste of necessity" wherein they come to prefer the
things they can afford.[16] For a variety of reasons—including affordability, shelf stability, coverage by food assistance programs like WIC, and
the costs of food spoilage and waste—low-income people in the United
States are more likely to eat processed foods with added preservatives
and less likely to be exposed to a range of fresh, highly perishable foods
(which also happen to be the foods dominant health discourses describe
as healthiest). These practical constraints on diet transform, over time,
into class cultural preferences that get imprinted on the body as *tastes*.[17]
Thus, when upper-middle-class women like Lara describe themselves
as having "always been a really healthy eater" and working-class women
like LaDonna self-identify as picky because "I really don't like fruits,"
they are describing a real cross-class difference in tastes. Mixed-class
women, especially those with middle-class cultural capital living on limited means, may feel particularly deprived by their economic circumstances: they have a taste for many foods and products that they cannot
afford to consume, and their distaste for the things they *can* afford is
viscerally uncomfortable.

The second important component of these class differences is the set
of symbolic rewards that women from different classes stand to reap
from adopting body- and health-centered self-identities. To truly live
up to the normative expectation that "good" modern subjects express
their values and identities through carefully cultivated body regimes, it
is not enough to do "the right thing" in one's reproductive body project.
Instead—as demonstrated by the middle- and upper-class women in
this chapter—one must express a personal devotion to healthism. These
women sometimes fell short in executing these practices. Nevertheless,
by performing their devotion to these ideals and expressing dismay if

they failed to achieve them, high-status women were able to shore up their identities as "good" mothers across a wide range of actual practices and to receive social recognition as worthy, health-focused subjects.

Mixed-class women had more work to do to reconcile their constrained choices with middle-class cultural norms for health, yet they, too, sought to establish their identities and social status through reference to their body projects. Women like Frankie Ford firmly differentiated themselves from the morally suspect health choices of low-income people (who used public benefits to buy "candy and Red Bull"), while Noura and others emphasized their middle-class tastes, lamenting their inability to consume products that would match their cultural values and self-identities.

For poor and working-class women, health-focused self-identity was a status trap. On one hand, these women *did* want to have good health and to ensure that their children were safe and well nourished. On the other hand, among women whose tastes and financial means made it difficult to consume health products and foods in normatively "good" ways, admitting that health and consumption practices should define their self-identity would mean admitting to having bad or failed identities. A handful of women did seem to accept that label—naming their choices as "lazy" or "hard-headed"—but most, particularly low-income women of color, responded to the demand for health-centric self-identities by *disidentifying* or by seeking out *alternative identities*. These responses demonstrated an unwillingness to play by the same status rules that middle- and upper-class women did (or, at least, a recognition that playing by those rules would set them up to lose). Instead, disidentifying with health norms and seeking out alternative, non-health-focused identities allowed these women to make pragmatic choices for their families' well-being without having to apologize for or express shame about their decisions.

5

# Rigid and Flexible Agency

*Navigating Bodily Change and Unpredictability*

Jen Vargas (biracial, twenty-nine, HH) was a graduate student of mixed white and Latina heritage who reflected on the many surprises that pregnancy and childbirth had brought her:

> I had read stuff, like that your hips would change; you might get stretch marks, and stuff like that. . . . But I didn't realize how long the [morning] sickness could get, and that was surprising. I didn't realize how tired I could be. And also, I was surprised when [my son] was first born and [I was having] the hormonal changes. . . . You know, [I heard] "You might feel kind of blue," but I could tell it was not my normal way of feeling. . . . It was weird. It was feeling a little more out of control. I'm usually pretty even most of the time, but feeling like I could cry or I could snap and get angry or something like that—it was feeling like I could at any moment fall apart.

As Jen vividly recounts, the lived experience of pregnant and postpartum embodiment is something that can catch even well-read mothers by surprise. The bodily changes that this period brings often come on suddenly and strongly, making them particularly noticeable. Jen's account of having postpartum "baby blues" (even, perhaps, postpartum depression) highlights the embodied alienation such changes can bring: on one hand, she was experiencing deep and intense feelings of sadness or anger; on the other hand, even in the midst of these strong feelings a part of her consciousness identified those feelings as uncharacteristic and, probably, brought on by hormones that were out of her control.

That pregnancy and childbirth cause changes in the body is no secret; nearly all mothers in my study described having some expectation of what was in store. But in their narrative retellings of how pregnancy, childbirth, or breastfeeding *felt*—accounts grounded in their own lived, bodily experience—most women described moments of confronting the unexpected. Typically introduced with a comment like "Nobody ever tells you" or "I had no idea," these stories highlighted moments when all the reading or received wisdom in the world was unable to prepare women for the often surprising, visceral lived experience of pregnant and postpartum embodiment. Women's narrative descriptions of how they responded in these moments provide the core data for this chapter.

Closely reading these narratives, this chapter delves into the intense bodily sensations, changing size and abilities, medical interventions, and more that women in my study experienced during and after pregnancy. For otherwise healthy, nondisabled adults, these sorts of rapid changes have the potential to unsettle one's understanding of self and self-efficacy: in particular, the expectation that our bodies will simply do our minds' bidding. Thus, I ask, How do changes in the body during or after pregnancy impact women's sense of agency? And how might differing social contexts, especially social class, affect women's responses to these bodily changes?

As mothers' narratives in the following sections will reveal, women across classes experienced many of the same physical changes and challenges, but they responded in markedly different ways. For middle- and upper-class women, these changes represented a body that was potentially out of control, and their narratives emphasized their quest to reassert control over their bodies through what I call "rigid agency." For poor and working-class women, a different form of agency, which I term "flexible agency," predominated. This latter group still made choices about their bodies and those of their children, but, in their own words, they were focused less on rigidly determining an outcome and more on flexibly negotiating different alternatives. While both approaches represent class-conditioned responses to situational context, I argue that one—rigid agency—falls more in line with classical conceptions of agency and full personhood, but the other—flexible agency—is better suited to helping mothers adapt and thrive through the bodily changes of pregnancy and postpartum embodiment.

## Embodying Agency

### Cultivating Control

Gender socialization in the United States (and elsewhere) teaches girls from an early age to work on their own bodies: to use diet and exercise to mold their bodies into a desirable shape; to learn to adorn and present those bodies in normatively feminine ways; and to manage their bodies as objects to be protected from harm. The body consciousness this work requires then forms the basis for women's reproductive body projects and risk-management efforts when they become mothers.

Underlying this work is the belief that the body is, as Susan Bordo calls it, "cultural plastic": an object that can be shaped and transformed through will power and hard work (and, perhaps, a couple of technolog-ical/medical interventions). In the words of the self-help advertisements Bordo studies, "The proper diet, the right amount of exercise and you can have, pretty much, any body you desire."[1] The notion of a "plastic," moldable body has not always existed. In the West, its rise corresponds with modernity and a sense of the world, more generally, as knowable and controllable. And despite its claims to universality—anybody can have any body one wants!—the notion of the endlessly modifiable body is premised on a number of exclusionary assumptions: that people will have the time and money to consume products that can aid in their body projects, and that their bodies are close enough to the norm—youthful, nondisabled, white—for such projects to make up the difference.

Despite these objections, the notion of the plastic body is ubiquitous in contemporary US culture. Gita Potter (Asian, twenty-seven, HL) of-fers one example of how this expectation plays out:

> After I was pregnant the first time, I still had like twelve pounds to lose, and so I did diet for a little while to be able to control my weight and get it back down to the level it was before my son was born. . . . My mom had me, and then never quite lost the weight from me, and then had my brother and never quite lost the weight from my brother, so she's got like sixty extra pounds just hanging around from that. I didn't want to feel that way, so it was important to me to try and get back. My goal was to be the same weight that I was [before I got pregnant].

Gita interpreted her mother's "extra" weight not as a common consequence of aging and bearing two children but as a failure of control. Driven by her mother's negative example, Gita determined that she needed to take charge of her body or she would end up, twenty-eight years later, still carrying the baby weight. I asked how that project had gone, and she responded, "It actually went really well! I had a friend and we did a challenge to lose eight pounds in eight weeks. And it was done by controlling the amount of calories that we ate. So every week we stepped on the scale. We had a blog that we blogged to each other about our progress and how we were doing eating that day. It was helpful to have a friend, and I ended up losing eleven pounds."

Gita's story of attempting to lose weight after a pregnancy is a familiar tale; of all the ways Americans attempt to change their bodies, intentional weight loss is probably the most popular—if not the most successful—pursuit. But this is also a narrative about *control*: Gita set a goal for her body, partnered with a friend to hold one another accountable, and restricted what she ate until she reached that goal.

A fixation on control was a common theme among mothers in my study, especially middle- and upper-class mothers. In describing their actions during pregnancy and thereafter, these women often spoke of exercising a rigid control over bodily outcomes and making thoroughly researched choices. Diane Sperry (white, thirty-seven, HH), already a mother of two, was in her third trimester of pregnancy when I interviewed her. Pregnancy had forced her to modify her strict exercise habits, first to accommodate the deep fatigue she experienced in her first trimester and then, at the time of our interview, to manage the discomfort of her growing belly. She explained, "I try to do yoga and go swimming a couple of times a week. It actually feels good, with the belly hanging down instead of pressing on everything." I asked how she expected things to continue through the remainder of her pregnancy, and she replied, "As long as you're not overdoing it and hurting yourself or really overdoing it and triggering contractions too early, there's really no reason to stop. The better shape you're in before labor, the better you'll get through labor." Having investigated the risks and benefits of prenatal exercise, Diane spoke confidently about her choice to stay active throughout her pregnancy; she believed that her efforts would facilitate a healthy, uncomplicated labor and delivery. She also described how these routines fit into her larger reproductive body project: "Having my first daughter sort of started me on this [health] journey. I didn't really care much about nutrition before she was born, but after, I started it. It's very important to me to try to prepare whole foods rather than prepackaged foods. I like to control the ingredients that I put into things. I spend a lot of time reading recipes and looking for different ideas. And I'm trying to exercise as much as I can." In addition to optimizing her own eating and exercise routines, Diane sought to instill these values in her kindergarten-aged daughter: she had recently enrolled her in a charter school that emphasized nutritious eating and offered daily yoga classes.

Diane's efforts to establish a consistent exercise routine and eating habits in her family—even in the face of significant fluctuations in her energy levels and physical ability—were common among middle- and upper-class women in my study. When faced with the changes of pregnancy and new motherhood, these women attempted to become experts in their new, unfamiliar bodies. They read about pregnancy extensively, buying such parenting tomes as *What to Expect When You're Expecting* and reading up on attachment parenting (a time-intensive approach to childrearing popular among many of my middle-class respondents). They supplemented this knowledge by searching the Internet for alternative explanations of and remedies for their bodily discomforts; they also posted questions to online message boards for new mothers. Finally, many went beyond their doctors' advice and conducted their own experiments to find the body-care and nutrition practices that worked best for their bodies.

Kimberly Peters (white, thirty, HH), described how listening to her body's tastes and feelings had led her to shop and cook in particular ways:

> I remember coming back from Brazil [where I lived for many years] and eating some of the foods, and tasting the preservatives in them, and just going, "What is this stuff? It doesn't taste right." . . . It just evolved from there. As I went to college, just realizing that when I ate certain things I didn't feel good after eating them. When I met my husband in college, he has said, in retrospect, that he used to deal with a lot of migraines, and then after we got married when we were out of college, he said, "The way you shop and the things that you eliminated from my diet got rid of the migraines."

Not only did Kimberly's reflexive attention to her shopping and cooking habits help her feel better but also, her husband believed that his health had benefited. Likewise, Juana Reyes (Latina, twenty-nine, HL) described how her experimentation with her diet led her to conclude that she was sensitive to carbohydrates: "I just started doing trial and error with my own body. I would eat something and then take note of what happened afterward. [Foods that made me feel sluggish] were always carbohydrates." Although most mothers heeded their doctors' advice, many, like Juana and Kimberly, also devoted time to experimenting and becoming experts on their own bodies. They noted how their bodies felt under varying conditions, then methodically adjusted their self-care practices like laboratory researchers until they reached the ends they sought.

### It's Good to Be an Agent: Self-Control and Social Status

In this way, higher-class mothers conceptualized their bodies as knowable, manageable, and subject to their own autonomous control. In other words, they exemplified classical notions of embodied *agency*. Historically, philosophers have conceptualized agency as "having the power to control, regulate, or rule over [one's] conduct. . . . The free agent's control standardly is described as an executive power, the power decisively to initiate courses of action in the face of available alternatives, the ability to do or not do."[2] Agency, in this view, is about having the power not only to exert one's will in the world but also to turn that will toward the control of one's own self "to master ignorant desires, powerful appetites, physical urges. . . . Being free has meant being capable of self-domination."[3] This notion of agency, at its root, fundamentally pits the human mind against its most animalistic bodily needs and urges. Correspondingly, the free, deliberate choices one makes regarding the use and cultivation of the body come to stand as evidence of one's *agency*, perhaps even one's moral worthiness.

Popular discourses in the West treat agency as a political and personal good. At the societal level, countries like the United States conceptualize freedom as "the absence of external obstacles to self-guided choice and action," celebrating policies that clear the way for personal liberty and agency.[4] At the individual level, being judged as sufficiently agentic—

rational, strong-willed, and with "the power decisively to initiate courses of action"—is often a precondition for legal personhood. People who are seen as having a limited capacity for agency, such as children or people with dementia, may be given *protection* instead of *freedom*; their legal status is that of dependents, not full citizens.

On its face, the link between bodily self-control and the rights and responsibilities of citizenship seems logical: If you cannot even govern yourself, how can you be trusted to govern others? Accordingly, maintaining control over one's body is a way to earn social esteem; losing control, by contrast, becomes a source of social shame. Yet, these social benefits and burdens to performing agency are not shared equally. Throughout Western history, the dualistic thinking involved in defining agency thus—as a victory of mind over matter, the successful control of an unruly body—has also defined some bodies as *more* unruly, more in need of being controlled.

*Gender* is one defining characteristic of those bodies. Both scientific and artistic discourses in the West portray female reproductive functions as illness, insanity, and even demonic possession: in other words, as a loss of control.[5] So-called "leaky" body functions like menstruation and lactation are viewed with suspicion and anxiety; women—but rarely men—are said to be at the mercy of their hormones, controlled by (rather than in control of) their bodies. Margrit Shildrick summarizes the gendering of embodiment thus: "Although both sexes clearly do have material bodies, only women, because of their more intimate association with reproduction, were seen as intrinsically unable to transcend them."[6]

Similar dualisms—between those in control of their bodies and those who are controlled by their bodies—also appear in discourses about *race*. Racist and colonial tropes have long perpetuated "racist ideology and imagery that construct non-European 'races' as 'primitive,' 'savage,' sexually animalistic, and indeed more *bodily* than the white 'races.'"[7] Sabrina Strings argues that the cultural linkage between fatness and Blackness reproduces this trope; the association of race with fat "entails the synchronized repression of 'savage' blackness and the generation of disciplined whiteness. The discourse of fatness as 'coarse,' 'immoral,' and 'black' worked to denigrate black women, and it concomitantly became the impetus for the promulgation of slender figures as the proper form of embodiment for elite white Christian women."[8] Racist and colonial discourses like this fixate on supposed differences in the morphology of different groups' bodies—especially differences in the size and appearance of genitalia and other sexual/reproductive features—to conclude that nonwhite others are less self-controlled, less agentic, even less than human. And as with gender dualisms, the effect of these discourses is to preserve white, male power: someone who is unable to control their own body requires someone—a master—to control it for them.

Finally, discourses of bodily control and lack of control align with cultural understandings of *class*. In describing aristocratic Victorian ideals of slenderness, Bordo writes, "A frail frame and lack of appetite signified not only spiritual transcendence of the desires of the flesh but *social* transcendence of the laboring, striving, 'economic' body."[9] Protestant moral values celebrated asceticism and the denial of bodily needs, such that "eating and drinking less became evidence of refinement, [as] too did the thinner figures such behavior produced."[10] And when Pierre Bourdieu outlined the cultural distinctions among classes in mid-twentieth-century France, he noted that class-based *tastes*, lifestyles, and material circumstances lead to the appearance of "class bodies" distinct from one another in shape, size, and mannerisms. He concluded that "the legitimate use of the body [according to upper-class standards] is spontaneously perceived as an index of moral uprightness, so that its opposite, a 'natural' body, is seen as an index of *laisser-aller* ('letting oneself go'), a culpable surrender to facility."[11]

In other words, under the ideologies that predominate in Western Europe and the United States, status and moral virtue adhere to those who can assert the right sort of control over their bodies. To act on one's appetites without restraint, or to otherwise display a "natural" body, is a signifier of being low-class: to lack taste. Thus, it stands to reason that individuals would benefit by using their bodies to demonstrate control, taste, and "moral uprightness"—in other words, to demonstrate bodily *agency*. And it stands to reason that their narrative accounts of their behavior would emphasize their claims to agency.

## Challenging and Extending Notions of Agency

Traditional definitions of agency that cast it as a universalizing question of "free" will elide the ways in which this capacity for action is tied to specific sociohistorical conditions; the ideal "free" subject who will exercise such agency is thus revealed as someone with a relatively high degree of social and bodily privilege: likely male, white, upper-class, and in good health (among other things). And yet, rather than appearing as the effect of the privilege these characteristics bestow, agency is more often portrayed as the cause, a moral and tenacious exercise of will power that legitimates one's social position.

When we look at the modes of action available to people in a broader range of bodies and social positions, how might our understandings of agency shift? Maternal bodies, for example, challenge the classical notion of agency as being seated in an autonomous, discrete self. Writes Iris Marion Young, "The pregnant subject . . . is decentered, split, and doubled in several ways. She experiences her body as herself and not herself."[12] Such was certainly the case for women like Lori Kent (white, twenty-nine, HH), who described the feeling of her child moving inside of her with nostalgia: "I would sit there in a meeting and I could count kicks. . . . It was nice; you had someone there with you, kind of. . . . When I went back to those meetings [after my baby was born] it just felt so lonely." Theresa Butler (white, thirty-three, HH) explained how pregnancy changed her consciousness of her body, adding, "I was having a phenomenological kind of awakening. Like, fully recognizing myself as a body in this world and that I'm making this other body inside of my uterus, right? Like I'm taking this little egg and this sperm—me, my body did that!—and just watching all the changes happen."

Classical definitions of agency claim that agents have the ability to distinguish between "aspects of oneself which are 'really' one's own . . . [and] those aspects of oneself and the world which are not."[13] For people like Lori and Theresa, though, pregnancy entailed a blurring of bodily boundaries: they experienced their bodies as both self and not-self. As we have already seen in chapter 2, maternal-embodiment norms demand that mothers learn to extend their consciousness so that they can notice and respond to the needs of bodies other than their own. But Theresa's and Lori's descriptions speak to more than just the responsibility to care for another; they illustrate the astonishment with which many mothers regarded the experience of holding another body within their own. Indeed, when Cass Blackwell (white, thirty-three, LH) states that "my body doesn't belong to me during these nine months," we can interpret her words both as reflecting a self-sacrificing ideology and as a factual description of the experience of living in a body that is shared with another.[14]

Alongside this critique of the bodily experiences that classical agency excludes is a second critique: that agency, as it is usually defined, relies on the Western, liberal preoccupation with autonomy and freedom of choice. Anthropologist Saba Mahmood asks what agency might look like if we do not start from "the belief that all human beings have an innate desire for freedom, [and] that we all somehow seek to assert our autonomy when allowed to do so."[15] Mahmood argues that while it is important to seek out the spaces in which marginalized people act, it is a mistake to look for agency only in moments of resistance (as she accuses many Western feminists of doing). Instead, she advocates for recognizing agency in the cultural and historical contexts within which marginalized people act: "If the ability to effect change in the world and in oneself is historically and culturally specific . . . then the meaning and sense of agency cannot be fixed in advance, but must emerge through an analysis of the particular concepts that enable specific modes of being, responsibility, and effectivity."[16] Agency, in this view, can take multiple forms: the actions we take to give our lives meaning or to make them livable may look like resistance to norms, but these may also involve learning how to inhabit or navigate between norms. A culturally literate analysis of agency, Mahmood adds, will focus not on determinations of whether particular individuals have agency but on the modes of action open to them within their cultural contexts and social locations. Thus, Mahmood redefines agency as a field of *socially structured capacities for action*: not agency versus structure, but agency always within structure, with no one assumed to be free from social constraints.

Feminist legal scholar Jennifer Denbow similarly focuses on the agency of women on the margins. Conventional wisdom holds that people who possess more choices—and fewer legal constraints on choice—will be empowered to act in accordance with their own interests and desires. But Denbow's examination of reproductive choice—namely, legal access to abortion—questions that assumption. Writes Denbow, "When a woman has the option to abort, she faces heightened responsibility . . . for the consequences of not exercising that option."[17] In other words, the availability of abortion may create pressure on women who are judged as unfit or unprepared for motherhood—those who are too young, too poor, and so on—to make the "responsible" choice to terminate their pregnancies.

In the sections that follow, I will heed these feminist scholars' work for thinking through the agency of women from varying racial/ethnic and class backgrounds. Like Mahmood, I aim not to judge individual women as having or lacking agency but to use these women's narratives to understand the choices they make and the ways that structural conditions—cultural and material differences in particular—shape the modes of agency available to them. And, following Denbow, I will ask whether having different choices about how to care for maternal and child bodies supports women's agency or, perhaps, constrains it: What obligations and expectations for action do such choices entail? In sum, to what extent do these women expect or desire control over the embodied processes of pregnancy, labor and delivery, and lactation? And how does such control factor in to women's own—and others'—judgment of their agency and moral status?

## Middle- and Upper-Class Mothers' Rigid Agency

For middle- and upper-class women, planning and control featured prominently in their narratives of maternal embodiment. In line with risk-avoidant and risk-assessing approaches to health described in chapter 3, many mothers laid out plans that would help them minimize the health risks they (or their children) faced. Lori Kent, speaking to me three months after the premature birth of her first child, was already looking ahead to her next pregnancy. She told me, "It's important to me to reduce my weight. Because the next time around when we have kids, I want to make sure that the pregnancy has every chance possible of going to term. And even if you're only slightly overweight that is a risk factor in terms of having a healthy pregnancy or not. I mean, some people can be grossly overweight and have wonderful pregnancies and people who are completely healthy have issues. But just to give it every chance, statistically, it makes more sense for me to be at my ideal weight."

Lori's eagerness to ensure a full-term pregnancy was understandable. Her newborn son had spent time in the NICU after she delivered him almost two months early, and it was a harrowing experience for Lori and husband. In Lori's telling, she had "been having a wonderful pregnancy. Every appointment had gone super well. I was able to walk my dog two miles a day." When her water broke just shy of the thirty-three-week mark, Lori was shaken, not just by the abrupt end to her pregnancy but also by the fact that what she had experienced as a healthy, "wonderful" pregnancy could go wrong so suddenly. Lori conceded that fat people (whom she called "grossly overweight") could have healthy, full-term pregnancies. But, despite the fact that she was already smaller than the average woman of her age, Lori resolved to lose weight before she conceived again: it felt like one thing she could control that might make a difference.

Like Lori, several women (primarily middle to upper class) spoke of their plans to manage their bodies to achieve sought-after pregnancy goals, claiming that they knew best what their bodies were capable of. MacKenzie Gervais (white, thirty, HH) was classified as "overweight" when she became pregnant but made drastic changes to her diet once she conceived. "I tried to eat cleaner. Stayed away from a lot of the heavily processed meats and stuff. Cut down on caffeine. Drank a ton of water. Tried to eat lean, clean food. . . . The last couple of weeks I had done a good job of maintaining weight—I only gained twenty pounds, which I thought was okay. My doctor said I would gain forty and I was determined to prove him wrong." Similarly, Masha Begovic (white, thirty-four, HH) added of her experience proving doctors wrong,

> I've disagreed with [the doctors] so many times that now I just rely on my research. . . . My doctor told me that I had a small frame and I would probably have to have a C-section; I wouldn't be able to have the twins the regular way and would probably have them at thirty-four weeks. . . . But my twins, actually, I carried to forty weeks and the only reason I had a C-section (and I *chose it* in the end) was because the first baby to come out [the fetus positioned lower, expected to be born first] was breech. So just to cut that risk I scheduled a C-section. I waited until the last possible week. And the twins were seven pounds each. . . . I just wanted to go back to the doctor and say, "Ha ha, I know my body better than you."

Masha and MacKenzie both resented medical professionals telling them what their pregnant bodies could—or could not—do. Their doctors' pronouncements sounded to Masha and MacKenzie as if they were questioning the women's ability to set and enact a goal: in other words, questioning their agency. Even when Masha had a C-section, she framed it to me as a *choice*; she had proven that her body was capable of carrying twins to term, and she elected to have a C-section because she was a responsible, risk-avoidant mother—not because she was unable to have a vaginal delivery (after all, she said to me, her first-born had "come out naturally").

Intensive planning and self-control in anticipation of childbirth and other events were common among the middle- and upper-class mothers I interviewed. So, too, were statements about *reasserting* control after an unexpected setback. Several mothers described the bodily aftermath of pregnancy as being mentally, as well as physically, uncomfortable. Charlotte Moran (biracial, thirty-two, HH) put it bluntly: "During pregnancy, I remember feeling out of control, like I had lost control of my body. The feeling after I had my baby of wanting to get back to a pre-baby body is totally about regaining control of this body that I feel I've lost control of." Misty Clifford (white, thirty-one, HH) added, "I was really anxious to get my body back. Because I enjoyed running . . . and physically exerting myself." And Alison Correia (white, twenty-nine, HH), an administrative assistant at a university, laughed as she recounted what her post-baby body felt like:

> Oh, I was a mess! I felt like I had no control over anything. There was no time. I had an infant and I went to work after she was born, working a full-time job and then coming home and trying to spend as much time with her as possible. . . . I was always under the impression that it [my body's messiness] was awful, but it was temporary. I knew that going in, so it was just a sacrifice I had to make. I just had to get through that initial stage of complete lack of control and then everything would even out.

For Alison, the cumulative demands of motherhood and full-time work meant that she had no time to pursue postpartum weight loss, get her hair cut, or even shave her legs. She concluded, "I didn't feel like I looked like myself anymore. I looked like some person had just taken over my body. But slowly, after the first year, things started to fall k into place." Alison framed her lack of control over her body as something she could anticipate—"I knew that going in"—and she also had faith that, if she was patient, she would be able to reclaim control eventually. Although femininity and sexual desirability played a part in women's post-baby body ideals, women like Charlotte, Misty, and Alison mainly emphasized the ties between bodily control and bodily integrity: feeling in control of their bodies meant feeling like *themselves*.

On the whole, middle- and upper-class mothers in my study approached their bodies as malleable projects to be worked on. They conducted their own research into self-care techniques and, as well-informed consumers choosing among a range of possible approaches, solicited advice from experts. Ultimately, in their eating habits during pregnancy, their efforts at breastfeeding, and their postpartum weight-loss regimens, these mothers modeled the sort of autonomous decision-making and goal-oriented behavior that I term, collectively, *"rigid agency"*—a mode of action that, despite feminist scholars' assertions that maternal embodiment inherently challenges traditional notions of agency, continues to reflect classical liberal ideals for the autonomous, self-sufficient agent.

## Poor and Working-Class Mothers' Flexible Agency

For well-off, well-educated mothers with the financial means to enact their plans (as well as the culturally conditioned expectation that they would be able to do so), narratives emphasizing *rigid agency* allowed them to assert their own foresight and efficacy, as well as to lay claim to a particularly recognizable form of agency. Yet these women's agency was made possible not only by individual determination but by structural conditions that supported and facilitated their choices. Poor and working-class mothers, who face a different set of social structural conditions, often lack access to the same modes of agency as the middle- and upper-class mothers described above. Instead, I will argue for a different mode of agency within this group: what I term *"flexible agency."* This form of agency arises from the realization that, when past experience has shown life circumstances to be out of one's control, one's time and energy may be better spent adapting to difficult conditions than continuing the stubborn pursuit of one set goal.

*Choosing Flexibility*

In contrast to the job flexibility that allowed many professional mothers to work from home with their newborns (and to enact particular body projects for themselves and their children), poor and working-class mothers in my study were often unmarried, working in low-wage positions or enrolled in work training programs. Tina Smith (Black, forty-one, LL) explained that her job stocking shelves at a grocery store made it nearly impossible to exclusively breastfeed, saying, "I can pump at work, but it's really not realistic to say that I'd be pumping every hour at work." Faced with the choice of either quitting her job to attempt breastfeeding at home as a single mother or switching her son to formula, Tina pragmatically opted for the latter. Furthermore, she insisted that she made a fully informed decision, saying, "I guess [WIC] figured you don't have the information, so they kind of push it [breastfeeding] on you. No, it's not that. It's a choice that I've made."

Tina's explicit invocation of the language of "choice" was rare among lower-income women in my study, but her acknowledgment of the limits she faced was common. Similar to middle-class women, many of the poor and working-class mothers I spoke to explained that they intended to breastfeed, but ran into pain or supply problems early on. As India Brown (Black, twenty, LL) described, "I wanted to breastfeed so bad. I was on board. Like, 'Breastfeeding is the way to go.' And then, when I had Elle, I could only breastfeed for about a week, maybe a week and four days, that's how long I breastfed her. It was just too painful for me. . . . Everybody had a lot of good things to say about breastfeeding. And I felt like it would have been the right way to go. But it wasn't right for me, at that particular time."

I asked India how she felt about this, and she responded, "I was kind of disappointed in myself. But you know? You can't do everything." As India's story shows, she knew that breastfeeding was supposed to provide the best nutrition for her child, and tried to do what she thought was best. Although she wished she could have continued to breastfeed, she refused to anguish over "failing." Shontel Sykes (Black, twenty, LL) also tried to breastfeed her son, but after a milk duct infection forced her to switch her son to formula temporarily, she decided to make the change permanent. For Shontel, who was sixteen when she had her first child, bottle feeding gave her the predictability and bodily freedom to continue her schooling and work part-time; importantly, it allowed her mother to share childcare responsibilities. Shontel had given breastfeeding her best shot, but when pain interrupted that plan, she was flexible enough in her plans to try formula, and she found that formula fit her needs even better.

Indeed, few of the WIC-eligible women in my study planned to offer formula from the outset. Most mothers had absorbed the lesson that breastmilk was best for their child, and sought to be good mothers by providing that. And, just like the middle- and upper-class mothers I interviewed, they sometimes ran into bodily limitations of supply, infection, or pain. The difference was in how mothers from the two groups responded to such difficulties. For middle- and upper-class mothers who had a strong cultural investment in achieving their goals and demonstrating their mastery of their bodies, breastfeeding troubles represented just one more physical hurdle standing between them and their aims; their response was to meet their breastfeeding goals (such as nursing for a full year) by pushing through and wrestling their unruly bodies into submission. In taking this approach, middle-class mothers acted with *rigid agency*. For poor and working-class mothers, however, *flexible agency* was the more practical approach. Faced with unanticipated problems in breastfeeding, these mothers were not so wedded to the "breast is best" ideology of their higher-income counterparts. Accordingly, they had less to lose by considering formula as a viable alternative. WIC-subsidized formula provided these women with a choice, and they took it—even though, according to the "breast is best" ideology, it was the wrong choice. Furthermore, they were more open to considering the positive implications that bottle feeding could have for their lives. Most WIC mothers in my study were unmarried, and switching their infants to formula allowed them to return to school or work, thereby enabling them to be better providers for their children.

These trends are shaped by race as well as class. According to Dawn Dow, Black women's own definitions of good motherhood emphasize "economic self-reliance, interdependent child care, and working as a duty of motherhood."[18] Dow observed these values in middle-class Black women but, given the legacy of racial wealth gaps in the United States, they were clearly shaped by communities' past experiences of financial precarity. Flexible agency and what Dow terms "integrative motherhood" are *adaptive*, especially for low-income mothers: these values and strategies prioritize family well-being writ large, including financial security and protection from racism, rather than narrowly focusing on physical health. Likewise, writes Jennifer Randles, the hegemonic "intensive mothering" ideologies common among white, class-privileged families operate "on a logic of maximizing children's potential and protecting their class status." In contrast, the "inventive mothering" practices of low-income mothers of color require "initiative and ingenuity" to compensate for what they cannot afford; such practices emphasize "maximizing children's access to basic needs and protecting their humanity."[19] Flexible agency allows low-income mothers to pursue healthful practices for themselves and their children while also protecting their self-worth when, at times, they must compromise their health goals to prioritize other family needs.

## Acknowledging Structural Limitations

When I asked Mercedes Diaz (Latina, nineteen, LL) about whether she had made any changes in how she cared for her body during pregnancy, she responded, "Not really, because I found out when I was four or five months [pregnant]. And I didn't gain any weight, whatsoever. I didn't have any cravings, any nausea, any symptoms at all. . . . I couldn't really tell, until just out of curiosity [I took a pregnancy test], and I was like, 'Crap, I'm pregnant!'" Mercedes' admission that the pregnancy took her by surprise was one way in which she and other poor and working-class mothers I interviewed framed their narratives very differently from those of middle-class mothers. Certainly, women of all classes sometimes found themselves unexpectedly pregnant, and those women made choices in the face of such surprises. However, middle- and upper-class mothers tended, in their self-narratives, to take credit for the choices they had made, while women like Mercedes tended to acknowledge the circumstances beyond their control.

Lacking control was a central theme in Mercedes' narrative. As Mercedes recounted her story, she reminded me of a pinball getting bounced around: due to her father's arrest and impending deportation, her mother and siblings had moved to live with relatives several hours away; Mercedes was left to choose between joining them or staying near her baby's father. Mercedes got engaged to her boyfriend and moved in with his family, but due to the economic downturn, work had dried up and they were facing foreclosure; Mercedes did not know where she would go if they lost the house. Despite these stressful circumstances, Mercedes endeavored to exercise and eat the sort of low-fat diet she believed would help her shed the "baby weight." Describing a friend who supported her in these efforts, Mercedes said, "I always go for walks with Anita. She tells me, 'Let's go to the gym.' But I'm not a member, so we just go for walks." Mercedes could not afford the gym fees, and even if she could, she would have had to find a babysitter for her son. Under those conditions, she attempted to get in shape as best she could. For Mercedes, agency meant working alongside significant structural forces—deportation proceedings, bankruptcy, an economic recession, and the physical aftermath of pregnancy—to make changes, however gradual, to improve her quality of life.

Mercedes' options for postpartum fitness were limited by her finances, a common theme among poor and working-class mothers I interviewed. Becky Baker (white, twenty-six, LL) explained, "I was feeling something was wrong with my body. I just wished I was not as big as I was, you know? . . . It was embarrassing to me. But it all comes with having a child, so you just learn to deal with it." Likewise, Shontel Sykes (Black, twenty, LL) reflected on her post-baby body and said, "It's not how I really want to look. I want something different, but everybody does." With this phrasing, Shontel simultaneously named and downplayed her dissatisfaction; her unspoken assertion was that deeply wanting something was not enough to achieve it, especially when she faced so many other demands on her attention. Sarah Evans (white, twenty-one, LL) described her efforts to balance weight loss, raising a child, and going back to school, saying, "It's hard to remember that you have to eat this and eat that. I can stay on a diet, it's just that when you get so busy . . . you forget." And Luz Flores (Latina, twenty-eight, LL) explained, "I feel fat. Because the babies are too little now, and I don't have time for doing more *ejercicio*." She added, "I have nine-month-old twins, and it's a twenty-four-hour job. Normally, I got to feed the babies, change the diapers. All night, no sleep too much. I drink like five or six cups of coffee every day to stay awake for the kids. . . . I'm so busy! And sometimes I have no time to eat. Or . . . I don't have time in the morning and I only eat at twelve, one, or later."

Stories about feeling tired, overwhelmed, and dissatisfied with one's body were not unique to low-income mothers. Parents of infants and toddlers routinely deal with sleep deprivation and a lack of time to care for their own bodies. And across classes, mothers I spoke to shared many of the same ideals for health and appearance. But when discussing these challenges, middle- and upper-class women were quicker to spell out how they planned to retake control. Poor and working-class mothers, in contrast, were more likely to stress accepting or adapting to their altered circumstances. What accounts for these differences?

Public discourses about poor and working-class women tend to frame them as making bad choices for their bodies, purportedly due to a lack of knowledge or strong cultural values. As Jennifer Denbow reminds us, the availability of choices does not merely expand opportunities for agency; it often entails holding people responsible for making the "right" choices (and applying scrutiny to poor and nonwhite people believed to be making the "wrong" choices).[20] Yet, my interviews with these women show that they shared many of the same values and hopes as middle- and upper-class mothers, but with far fewer resources for attaining those goals, and with greater material limitations on their available options. It is important to keep these structural constraints in mind when examining poor and working-class women's self-care practices. However, such structural analyses do subjects a disservice if they do not also consider other modalities of action besides the autonomous, control-focused agency that typifies my high-status respondents. In the face of uncertain life circumstances, poor and working-class women I interviewed juggled their responsibilities, often very deftly. When something did not go according to plan, they responded with *flexible agency*—that is, they quickly adjusted their course of action, letting go of one expectation and moving on to the next, working within constraints to effect whatever change they could in themselves and the world around them. In this way, their stories reveal the particular mode of action—the *flexible agency*—that is commonly available to poor and working-class US mothers.

## The Best-Laid Plans: Agency in Response to Adversity

The terms "rigid agency" and "flexible agency" characterize the general patterns of action (and justification for action) I observed among middle/upper-class and poor/working-class women, respectively, but they were not absolute. In particular, HH women often encountered bodily limitations that they could not plan and work their way through; in such cases, they needed to develop greater flexibility, but rarely did they find it easy.

### "I was going crazy trying to do it all": Rigid Agency and Unruly Bodies

Florida mother Sonia Gallo (Latina, thirty-five, HH) shared a common story of breastfeeding difficulties, recounting, "It started getting hard, because I was having production issues. And then I was having clogging ducts, and then I was getting mastitis. I'm trying to pump and the baby's screaming. . . . I was going to see a lactation consultant and taking natural herb supplements to try to produce more, to try to prevent clogged ducts. An array of different things. And I was going crazy, trying to do it all and wasn't enjoying it. It wasn't a happy moment. [My solution] should have probably been formula a lot sooner." Sonia eventually reconciled herself to offering formula, but she struggled through several miserable months before she accepted that she should. Gita Potter (Asian, twenty-seven, HL) recalled,

> I don't think people were realistic with me about hard it was going to be. . . . It took a lot of time and it was painful. I associated being able to breastfeed successfully with being a good mother, and not being able to breastfeed successfully with not being a good mother. And when I wasn't able to produce enough milk, even after I was taking all these supplements and everything . . . I had to supplement with formula. I remember feeling like I was not going to be a good mom, because I couldn't breastfeed my child solely.

The experience of having difficulty breastfeeding is not particular to any one class; Gita's response, however, reflected her middle-class upbringing (rather than her current low socioeconomic status, due to being a stay-at-home mother while her husband was a medical student). Steeped in the biomedical vision of a "plastic body," and confident in her meritocratic belief that self-discipline and hard work could deliver the results she desired, Gita had no notion that her body might evade her control. Like Sonia's, Gita's body forced her to confront the limits of her control and accept, however painfully, an alternative approach to infant feeding.

Unlike Gita and Sonia, Lara Noble (white, forty, HH) had no issues with production, but instead was thrown for a loop when her four-month-old went on a nursing strike. Lara, who had cherished an extended breastfeeding relationship with her first child, was heartbroken: "I actually went back to therapy for the first time in years over this, because it was so devastating to me not to be able to nurse her. . . . I've made peace with it, but it's hard. There's a piece of me that wants to have a third child just so I can have this nursing relationship again." Lara was not the only woman to describe the bodily upheavals of maternal embodiment as psychologically harmful. Cass Blackwell (white, thirty-three, LH) recounted her profound disappointment when the vaginal delivery she had hoped for turned into a scheduled C-section, saying,

> I kept trying to will my body to go into labor, and it just didn't happen. . . . The C-section, the whole thing was just scary and frightening. I'd never had any major surgery before in my life. They put you on this table that's like a sacrificial cross or something, and then they have to tilt the table so you're at an angle for them to do what it is that they're doing. . . . It's just totally surreal. So it was not the way I had envisioned it happening. [My daughter] was still absolutely beautiful, but it was a bit traumatic for me. It definitely was not my expectation for what my perfect birth would have been.

Cass attributed her postpartum depression to the trauma of her daughter's birth; while she was glad her daughter was born safe, she also found it hard to get past her disappointed hopes and plans.

*"Having a plan and going into it mindfully": Navigating Rigidity and Flexibility*

Some middle-class mothers anticipated the need for flexibility. For example, Bree Turner (white, thirty-three, HH) consciously cultivated flexibility by enrolling in prenatal "mindfulness" classes, which she described thus: "It's not trying to control every aspect of your child's birth. [It's] having a plan and going into it mindfully." The birth plan Bree developed was a document she and many other middle-class mothers crafted in hopes of retaining a measure of control over one of the most potentially out-of-control-seeming experiences of maternal embodiment: childbirth. Social critic Naomi Wolf describes the promises and pitfalls of this document: "Hospitals and obstetrical practices that deal with demanding clients such as our educated cohort encourage couples to write such a plan, as it gives us a sense of consumer choice. We are not told outright that it is hospital protocols that determine what will happen in the course of delivery, usually regardless of what one's plan might say. . . . The joke is that you would believe that you have any power in the hospital to change the outcome."[21]

Many middle- and upper-class mothers I interviewed did extensive research about how to have the "best" childbirth experience. "Natural" (nonmedicated, vaginal) delivery was often idealized, both for its supposed health benefits and for the greater degree of control it allegedly offered mothers over their bodies. These women also sought to retain control in childbirth through their choices as consumers of care: many preferred to staff their deliveries with midwives (believed to impose fewer unnecessary medical interventions) and doulas (nonmedical childbirth attendants who support a pregnant person during labor and delivery, helping to advocate for their plans in medical settings). Despite these well-laid plans, however, childbirth often did not go as expected. Complications in pregnancy sometimes foiled mothers' hopes for home births, and difficult labors led women to accept labor-inducing drugs and painkillers that they had wished to avoid.

Bree, for example, ultimately assented to her obstetrician's suggestion that she accept epidural anesthesia for the pain. She credited this adaptability to her prenatal cultivation of mindfulness: "The one thing I learned . . . was, you need to be flexible. And that if you hold on to something rigidly—anything—and then it goes differently, it's very hard to get over that." Essentially, Bree had incorporated a small measure of flexible agency into her rigidly agentic outlook, using it to help her negotiate not financial limitations on her choices but bodily ones. However, lest this perspective be taken as passivity and inaction, Bree carefully reframed it as evidence of her intentional, agentic preparation for becoming a mother.

Amanda Katz (white, thirty, HH) likewise worked to find a sense of control in an out-of-control situation. She explained, "I did have a birth plan, but it went all out the window." Five weeks before her due date, Amanda went into precipitous labor, which came on suddenly and progressed rapidly. A nurse herself, Amanda had not planned on having any medical interventions, but once she was in labor, she agreed to an epidural. She explained, "It was so scary to give birth that early. . . . I felt so out of control with what was happening that having the epidural gave me some feeling of being in control because I wasn't focused on the pain. I was focused on why we were here." Although Amanda's labor and delivery did not go according to plan—in retrospect, she called the process "traumatic"—she reframed her choices as giving her control and helping her prepare for the birth of her son.

Likewise, Suzanne Walsh (white, thirty-five, HH) had planned on having a "natural" childbirth. However, after her labor stalled, her caregivers recommended an epidural and Pitocin, a synthetic hormone similar to oxytocin, to induce contractions. Suzanne described the absolute loss of control she felt: "I had back labor, which is where she is coming up against your spinal path. So that was really, really brutal. That was the most out-of-body experience I'd ever had in my life. I felt like a feral animal. I can't describe it; I can't put it into words. It's not human." Faced with this level of pain, she assented to the doctors' proposal for anesthesia. She told me, "At one point I was like 'Giddy-up! Giddy-fucking-up. I'm in this. My plan is so out the window.' And I was fine with it. Whatever is happening is happening." Hours later, the medications began to wear off, and she grudgingly agreed to a second epidural. Even as she consented, Suzanne harbored a secret wish to regain bodily control: "I had a thought in my head: 'I'm not going to get [the epidural] again.' I had a lot of faith in my body. So by five p.m., just as the anesthesiologist was walking into the room, the nurse checked me again. . . . I was at ten [centimeters—fully dilated and ready to give birth]. Just as this dude [the doctor] was walking in the room. And I was like, 'I'm not getting an epidural!'" Suzanne temporarily relinquished her rigid control over her body, a flexibility that gave her respite from the pain of childbirth and allowed her to rest. However, the familiar urge to control her body reappeared before long, and Suzanne completed her labor "naturally," thereby reclaiming the sense of self with which she identified. Few middle- or upper-class women shifted between flexible and rigid agency so quickly, but many did seek to reassert the type of rigid self-control traditionally associated with agency soon after giving birth, or, as Bree did, to narratively frame their flexibility as part of a calculated plan for self-improvement.

By contrast, stories about control and loss of control in the delivery room were practically nonexistent among lower-income mothers in my study. I should note that my initial interview guide did not include questions about labor and delivery, because I aimed to study the practices of self-care these women cultivated in their day-to-day lives, rather than the acute conditions they faced during labor. Nonetheless, childbirth became an emergent category in my analysis as numerous middle- and upper-class mothers volunteered their stories; clearly, for these women, it posed a critical challenge to preconceived notions about bodily integrity and self-control. As such stories make plain, childbirth (and, to some extent, breastfeeding) is among the most idealized venues for self-management, but it is also an arena in which bodily self-determination is most elusive. Both the physical realities of childbirth, which sometimes necessitated medical intervention, and the legal and medical norms observed by hospitals structured a setting in which middle- and upper-class mothers were less likely to have the control they desired. As a result, these women found themselves forced to adopt a measure of flexibility (which, to some, felt like a *loss* of agency and a threat to self-identity).

### "If I can't handle it, I'm not going to be mad at myself": Flexibility and Unpredictability in Maternal Embodiment

Poor and working-class mothers took a different approach to the unpredictable nature of pregnancy and childbirth. For one thing, relatively fewer of these mothers cited specific plans for birth or shared stories about their deliveries. Some, like mixed-class Ji-Eun Park (Asian, thirty-five, HL), explained that going into her first two deliveries, "I didn't have any plan, actually." Others, like Becky Baker (white, twenty-six, LL), had some notion of what to expect, but without much sense that it was under their control. She explained, "People tell you all the stuff that's going to happen after the baby, while you're giving birth. . . . It got me scared! I was super-scared when I heard it. I was like, 'All this stuff is happening? Holy cow!' . . . And then it happened, and I was like 'Oh my gosh! This is horrible!' Breastfeeding, in general, is a horrible experience. It hurts so bad!" For Becky, childbirth and breastfeeding did not feel like processes she had the power to direct; rather, they were painful, frightening experiences that happened to her. Even with advance warning about what to expect, Becky summarized the experience as "horrible."

Some scholars have argued that poor and working-class women do not *desire* control over pregnancy and childbirth. According to Margaret K. Nelson, working-class women "are less likely than middle class women to favor a natural childbirth, to plan for each stage of the birth process, and to prefer giving birth without medical intervention. During the birthing itself, working class women experience more medical intervention and less active involvement in the birth process."[22] Anthropologist Ellen Lazarus found similar patterns according to class. Whereas middle-class mothers in her study sought to control their pregnancies and deliveries, often by recruiting a trusted physician as their advocate, "Poor women neither expected nor desired control but were more concerned with continuity of care."[23]

The experiences of women in my study tell a rather different story, and suggest alternate explanations. First, a number of low-income mothers *did* make plans for childbirth, perhaps due to information about alternatives to medicalized childbirth becoming more widespread thanks to the popularity of Ricki Lake and Abby Epstein's 2008 documentary, *The Business of Being Born*, and books like Ina May Gaskin's *Spiritual Midwifery*.[24] Dani Hahn (white, twenty-four, LH) was a mixed-class mother who told me about how she planned for a "natural" water birth but ended up needing a last-minute Caesarian section, commenting, "I was kind of bummed about that. . . .'Cause I had a plan." I asked why she had hoped to deliver in the midwife-run birth center, and she responded, "I have a really high pain tolerance, so I wanted to test myself and see. You know, if I can't handle it, I'm not going to be mad at myself. I could ask to go to the hospital." Even though Dani was frustrated about her lost opportunity to "test" herself in this way, her subsequent comments revealed that she maintained a flexible mindset and an openness to changing the plan as needed. Grace Kellogg (white, twenty, LL) had a similar story. Grace lived in the same region as Dani, which was home to a nationally recognized midwifery school and birth center. Like Dani, Grace described her wish for a water birth staffed by midwives; she added that "I thought it would be so cool without medicine or anything because it's my first pregnancy. I don't need medicine. I can do this!" But, also like Dani, Grace encountered complications toward the end of her pregnancy that made unmedicated childbirth riskier. She was disappointed by this turn of events, but also deeply appreciative of the obstetrician who delivered her son: "She was really good. I didn't want the episiotomy. [I said,] 'If I'm going to tear, I'm going to tear.' But in the heat of it all, she's like, 'He's not going to come out.' So I was like, 'Just do whatever you got to do, I just want my baby.'" Grace's doctor proceeded with the episiotomy (a small, front-to-back incision made to enlarge the vaginal opening during childbirth). Grace, laughing as she recounted the story, concluded, "I think it was like two pushes and he was out. . . . His head was too big!" In the physical details of their births, Dani and Grace's stories are comparable to those of middle- and upper-class mothers who tried to have "natural" deliveries but ran into health complications that elicited medical intervention. But unlike the many high-status respondents who lingered over what they experienced as "trauma" resulting from their loss of control, women like Dani and Grace described those moments with relative resilience: frustration, perhaps, but also acceptance and an ability to move on.

Second, for the majority of the low-income women I interviewed who did not voice strong preferences about their deliveries—seeming to support Nelson's and Lazarus's findings that working-class women "neither expected nor desired" control—a closer examination of the structural influences on their "choices" is warranted. In 2010, approximately 45 percent of all births in the United States were covered by Medicaid, a figure that included most of the low-income women in my study.[25] As a state-administered public health insurance program for low-income people, Medicaid does not prioritize customer choice in its maternity-care options. State Medicaid programs frequently limit the specific types and frequency of services they will cover to reduce their costs. Furthermore, some states only permit Medicaid funds to be used for hospital births, refusing coverage for the less medicalized options of birth centers or home births. Khiara Bridges describes how low-income mothers in this system experience "excessive medicalization" relative to privately insured mothers-to-be.[26] Such medicalization treats poor and working-class women's bodies as inherently higher risk and in need of firm oversight by medical professionals, while offering them less discretion to select the birthing options best suited to their own bodies and comfort.

Medicaid-enrolled women's healthcare choices are further curtailed by the unwillingness of some healthcare providers to accept Medicaid patients. As a rule, Medicaid reimburses providers at a lower rate than do private health insurance plans, which makes Medicaid patients less profitable to treat. It follows that many hospitals and healthcare practices will not accept Medicaid-enrolled patients: a 2019 report found that only about 71 percent of physicians surveyed said they would accept new patients with Medicaid, compared to 90 percent who said they would accept new patients with private insurance.[27] Under this system, pregnant patients insured by Medicaid have fewer choices in where to seek care, and those options that do exist are often worse in quality, resulting in worse outcomes relative to the types of providers and services available to privately insured patients.[28] As Katherine Johnson and Richard Simon put it, women who experience racial and/or class disadvantage "receive less *and* more childbirth interventions—both of which appear to be out of sync with their birthing preferences."[29]

Given the restrictions imposed upon them, it stands to reason that low-income women might not invest too much time in developing a birth plan, especially one that limits medical interventions: What is the point, when one's health providers or insurer might not even allow one to enact that plan?

One additional reason why low-income women, especially women of color, might hesitate to make too many demands on their providers is the abiding presence of racism and racially disparate outcomes in healthcare. Black women in the United States are between three and four times more likely to die from pregnancy-related causes than white women (a phenomenon known as the Black maternal mortality crisis), and Black infants are more than twice as likely to die as white infants.[30] Similar disparities in maternal and infant mortality exist for Native American and Alaska Native populations.[31] Consistent with racism elsewhere in the system, Black and Native women are at risk for having their concerns overlooked by healthcare providers, who are more likely to see them as exaggerating pain or discomfort (see, for example, the near-death experience of tennis superstar Serena Williams in 2017 after doctors disregarded her reports of postpartum complications). Accordingly, these women may, whether consciously or unconsciously, try to ration the demands they make on their providers, so that when they do have a serious health concern, they are less likely to be dismissed as "difficult" or "needy."

In summary, poor and working-class women in my study were significantly less fixated on controlling each step of their pregnancies and deliveries. That flexibility, I argue, is adaptive: low-income women know that the systems they rely on for care are not usually set up to prioritize customer choice, and for Black and Indigenous women in particular, it can be a struggle even to get acute health concerns taken seriously. Under such conditions, women tend to express a form of agency that centers flexibility and resilience: sometimes making plans, but also being ready to adapt when things do not go according to plan. Sometimes the barriers to having the birth—or pregnancy, or breastfeeding experience—one desires are structural, such as a system that medicalizes pregnancy and childbirth generally and for low-income women especially. At other times, the barriers are simply bodily: a stalled labor or breech position that will not progress without medical intervention, or a low supply of breastmilk that no amount of pumping or ingesting supplements will resolve. Low-income women's *flexible agency* equipped them to deal with both.

In contrast, middle- and upper-class women's *rigid agency* was grounded in a deep faith in both their own bodies' abilities and, at times, the ability of conventional or alternative medicine to deliver the outcomes they desired. If low-income women's experiences had taught them to expect little control over their own care (and little responsiveness from providers), higher-class women's past experiences had taught them that there was no barrier they could not overcome if they invested enough will power, effort, or money. That expectation was born out of a class-conditioned sense of entitlement to professionals' time and personal attention, as well as the "Type A," achievement-oriented identities that many professional women cultivated.[32] This expectation of control, however, could sometimes pose a problem. When some element of maternal embodiment did not go according to plan, middle- and upper-class mothers often fought to retain control over the process; their response, grounded in *rigid agency*, often left them emotionally distraught over their so-called failures, resentful of healthcare providers, or even resistant to health-preserving interventions.

My intention here is not to diminish the real sense of loss that some women felt when things did not go according to plan, nor do I wish to suggest that laboring people should have no say in what happens to their bodies—obviously, they should. And when it comes to the healthcare systems through which we access care—public or private insurance, higher or lower levels of medical oversight and intervention—every pregnant and laboring person deserves responsive, clear communication about their options for care. Recent efforts to bring midwifery and doula services to low-income, racial/ethnic minority, and incarcerated populations in the United States represent an important step toward expanding access to such care.

But I would argue that the neoliberal expectation that our bodies should be fully under our control, and the belief that such control is possible, sets many of us up for profound disappointment when, sooner or later, our bodies have other ideas. Given the extent to which childbearing and childrearing entail circumstances beyond our control—and, thus, a need for flexibility—might poor and working-class women have an easier adjustment to some aspects of motherhood? Furthermore, how might those women's structural location enable them to more fully embrace the alternative forms of agency—the blurring of bodily boundaries as well as the need for flexibility—made visible by maternal embodiment?

## Conclusion

Women I spoke to described numerous paths to motherhood that included infertility, miscarriages, and unintended pregnancies;

pregnancy symptoms ranging from minor nausea to full-body rashes; and deliveries where everything or nothing went according to plan. While mothers sometimes regarded their bodies' life-giving abilities with wonder, when difficulties arose, those same bodies also presented a challenge to women's sense of agency and control. This was particularly the case for young, relatively healthy first-time mothers who, through past successes with dieting and other body projects, took their bodily self-control for granted. Faced with maternal bodies that sometimes eluded their control, middle- and upper-class women, in particular, struggled to regain control or to come to terms with their lack of control.

This phenomenon is not limited to mothers. Scholars of disability and chronic illness have noted that other changes in the body's health and abilities—as well as stresses on interpersonal relationships as a result—can cause "biographical disruption" in people with disabilities.[33] But such disruptions do not affect everyone equally; different groups of people have markedly different degrees of ease when adapting to a newly acquired disability. Girls and women, for example, typically adapt to chronic illnesses and impairments more readily than do men and boys.[34] This gap is due to gender norms that link masculinity with bodies that are active, productive, independent, and virile, while feminine embodiment already emphasizes the body's vulnerability and need for care. Furthermore, scholars of aging have found that people with positive perceptions of aging—that is, people who do not equate the changing capabilities of old age with a loss of identity and purpose—have significantly longer lifespans, even after controlling for differences in baseline health.[35]

Maternal embodiment differs from these conditions in that it involves a temporary, rather than a permanent, change in the body's functioning. Indeed, the proposition that pregnancy should be considered as a type of disability is controversial, and few pregnant people would self-identify as disabled on the basis of pregnancy alone. But pregnancy and other stages of maternal embodiment nevertheless force subjects to confront some of the ableist assumptions we are taught about the body: namely, that the able body "can be trained to do almost anything; it adjusts to new situations" and the corollary view that "disability can be overcome through will power or acts of the imagination."[36]

For mothers who ran up against the limitations of their ability to train and control their bodies or to overcome setbacks, class cultural differences mediated their responses. Middle- and upper-class mothers typically voiced determination to reassert control, epitomized by Charlotte Moran's statement that "the feeling after I had my baby of wanting to get back to a pre-baby body is totally about regaining control of this body that I feel I've lost control of." Class-privileged women who failed to regain control used words like "heartbreak" and "trauma" to describe the mental and emotional costs of that struggle. Rigid agency, for these mothers, can be a source of strength, but it can also be brittle: when it gives out, the fallout can be destructive and hard to heal.

In contrast, poor and working-class modes of agency tended more toward *flexibility*: not an absence of hopes and goals for one's body but a greater ability to adapt to unexpected stresses and barriers. Low-income women who faced challenging bodily setbacks during and after pregnancy were not happy about these circumstances—they frequently voiced negative emotions like disappointment or frustration—but they also tended to process these feelings with resilience, finding ways to accept what had happened and to move on.

Past research on disability and aging suggests that people who are able to adapt to changing bodily needs and functionality and incorporate these changes into their self-concept will have not only better psychosocial outcomes but also better physical health in the long term. Such adaptability often varies along gender lines (where women/femininity have greater capacity for change). This project is the first that I know of to examine *class* differences in adaptability. All told, this suggests that poor and working-class mothers' flexible agency with regard to their changing bodies and abilities may be a powerful resource for both mental and physical health; furthermore, it suggests that middle- and upper-class efforts to "take charge" of the body may be more harmful than they are empowering.

# 6

## Care Work as Status Work

### *The Child's Body as a Site of Social Reproduction*

Cass Blackwell was a soft-spoken, thirty-three-year-old white mother of one whom I interviewed at her home in Florida. It was the kind of suffocatingly hot, humid August day that drove locals into the comfort of their air-conditioned homes, and Cass had invited another mom—Emily Fischer, a new friend from her postpartum-depression support group—to join us for a combined interview and play date. Their three-month-old daughters, born about two weeks apart, ate and napped while we spoke, and I asked the two women about their eating habits and what they hoped to eventually teach their children. Cass replied first: "Right now, [we eat] just whatever I can manage. And as she gets older, I'm sure that will change, because I don't want her eating junk food and things like that, like Halloween candy. I think there's an age where that's appropriate, but she's just so little right now, that I don't want her to learn bad habits right off the bat. So as she gets bigger and starts eating solids and being able to sit at the table with us and eat a meal, I think our eating habits will change for the better. So—" Cass began to elaborate on the challenges to eating healthily that she and her husband faced in the present, but Emily cut in, announcing,

I don't eat diet food, ever. EV-ER. If it's not supposed to be sugar-free and it is, I don't eat it. If it's not supposed to be fat free and it is, I don't eat it. And that was one thing that I discovered [when I lived] in Switzerland. Because they don't have the low-fat products. There is no skim milk. It does not exist in Switzerland. So we just ended up eating real food, and we felt so much more satiated that I ended up eating less overall. If I can have a small portion of real ice cream instead of a large portion of low-fat frozen yogurt, 'cause I'm trying to get that *feeling*. . . . You know, we don't do that [eat diet food] in our house. I don't do NutraSweet at all. I don't drink diet pop. It's all real food. I just try not to go crazy with it. And I just want to teach my daughter, you can eat whatever you want in moderation. It's not about never having sweets. It's not about never having carbs. If you have a well-rounded diet, then the occasional cheesecake is not going to be a problem.

The visions of healthful eating that Cass and Emily laid out were distinct. While mixed-class Cass focused on avoiding "junk" foods like candy and prioritizing family meals, Emily (white, thirty-one, HH) instead spoke scathingly about so-called diet foods, many of which are heavily processed, and voiced a preference for eating what she called "real" foods in moderation. These two attitudes represent different iterations of diet marketing in the United States. In the 1990s, low-fat processed foods like Snackwell's fat-free cookies reigned, only to be eclipsed first by the low-carbohydrate diets (such as the Atkins diet) of the early 2000s and then by the movement toward "real" (minimally processed) or "slow" foods led by critic Michael Pollan (*In Defense of Food*, 2008), who declared that people should eat foods that "our great grandmothers would recognize as food" and that healthful eating should follow a simple motto: "Eat food. Not too much. Mostly plants." Emily's insistence on eating "real food" marked her as being in touch with the most up-to-date dietary trends when I interviewed her in 2010; Emily also tied her food values to the time she and her husband had spent living in Switzerland, asserting a sort of elite cultural knowledge as a result of her cosmopolitan lifestyle.[1] Cass's focus on avoiding candy and "junk food," in contrast, represented a more general (and somewhat dated) approach to discerning "good" from "bad" foods.

The differing frames that Cass and Emily used to think about healthful eating reflected class trends I saw across women in Florida and California. Cass came from solidly blue-collar origins: her father had retired from the navy to sell air-conditioning equipment when she was a child, and her mother worked part-time from home as a telemarketer. Neither of her parents had gone to college, and Cass herself had attended but not graduated. In recent years, though, Cass and her husband's combined incomes had lifted them into a tenuously middle-class existence in the relatively low-cost-of-living area of Florida where they resided. Emily, on the other hand, had followed in both of her parents' footsteps to earn a master's degree in education and pursue a career as a teacher. Emily's parents were not wealthy—they taught in public high schools—but she did acquire high-status cultural capital as a result of her and her parents' education. Emily's husband, on the other hand, brought a substantial amount of inherited family wealth to supplement their household income, and his work as a postdoctoral researcher gave them the opportunity to travel around the world. Thus, although Cass and Emily shared many things—first as white girls growing up in the same midwestern city in the 1980s, then as first-time moms who both struggled with postpartum depression—their educational and material differences placed them in markedly different social spheres. The two had connected in spite of their differences, but their friendship was un-usual among women I studied.

On the day I interviewed them, the choices Cass and Emily faced when it came to nurturing their infant daughters' bodies were relatively simple: Emily offered a combination of pumped breastmilk and infant formula, and Cass opted for formula alone. But even three months post-partum, both women were already looking ahead to how they would endow their children with healthy habits and values to last a lifetime. This chapter examines the divergent values and strategies women of dif-ferent classes adopted as they set about passing on health and body-care ideologies to their children. Mothers of higher and lower statuses tended, like Emily and Cass, to diverge on the criteria they used to judge particular foods and health practices as "good" or "bad." Poor and working-class mothers were more likely to teach their children specific guidelines for healthful habits, while middle- and upper-class mothers emphasized teaching kids to become informed consumers and early adopters: the kind of people who can read food labels, think critically about health trends, and adapt to new information and guidelines as they develop. And while class-privileged mothers recognized the so-cial benefits that could accrue to their children from cultivating diverse bodily tastes and knowledges, low-income mothers—especially certain women of color—more often focused on making children's bodies pre-sentable and respectable.

Mothers across classes invested significant energy into teaching children these lessons about health and body care as a labor of love: they spoke of wanting children to cherish their own bodies in ways that mothers often struggled to do for themselves; they sought to protect children from ill health or the dangers of drugs and violence; and they dreamed of a future where children could experience their bodies as powerful, capable, and sacred. At the same time, I argue that mothers' efforts are also a form of *status work*, reproducing class-differentiated patterns of body care—often, but not always, unconsciously. Previous scholarship has studied the ways in which class cultural differences in parenting styles place children on different social tracks as early as elementary school. Here, I argue that those disparities begin earlier still: in toddlerhood, infancy, and even in utero. Social status is thus both a *contributor* to class differences in body care and a *consequence* of those differences.

## Setting the Stage: Social Reproduction and Family Life

Mothers who seek to pass on class-specific knowledges and advantages are taking part in what social scientists call "social reproduction," transmitting their own social status, culture, and resources to their children. In cultures with strictly enforced caste systems or other formal hierarchies, social reproduction is near absolute: the children of peasants become peasants, for example, and only children born into a priestly caste can become priests. In other cultures, individuals may find more opportunities for upward (or downward) mobility relative to their parents' status. In the United States, as in many other highly developed capitalist democracies, parental status is *highly predictive*, but not *determinative*, of children's eventual social status. The children of college-educated, white-collar professionals are most likely to become white-collar professionals themselves (especially if they are white); the children of low-wage manual laborers are most likely to hold similar jobs when they enter the workforce (especially if they are Black).[2] The reasons for this are mainly structural: public schools are funded by local property taxes, meaning that children from wealthier (often racially segregated) neighborhoods have access to better-funded schools; college is both expensive and essential for getting a "good" job; and young adults often locate internships and career opportunities through their families' social networks. Through these and other factors, children of high-status parents have disproportionate access to the kinds of economic and social resources that will help them attain educational and occupational success. Yet, because a significant minority of individuals *do* move up or down relative to their parents' status, many parents, whether consciously or unconsciously, feel pressure to ensure their child's future status: to help them achieve upward mobility or, in the case of high-status families, to fend off competitors and safeguard their child's elite status. The particular form of caregiving work they perform to secure their children's future status I call "*status work.*"

Previous scholarship on early childhood socialization and social reproduction has tended to focus on schooling: What kinds of educational opportunities do children from different backgrounds have access to, and how well do parents prepare children to take advantage of those opportunities? Michèle Lamont and Mario Luís Small argue that "middle and upper-middle class adults (professionals and managers) pass on advantages to their children, mostly by familiarizing them with cultural habits and orientations valued by the educational system."[3] These cultural habits and orientations, also known as "cultural capital," allow children with the right kinds of habits to signal their fitness to teachers (and, later, employers). For example, children who demonstrate an ability to sit quietly, look attentive, and speak calmly and confidently to adults are signaling that they are "good" students; those who fidget, speak out of turn, or observe without vocally participating are more likely to be labeled as potential "problem" students in need of discipline or remedial education. Annette Lareau describes how these traits develop in the context of class and family life:

> [Middle-class families] are committed to child-rearing strategies that favor the individual development of each child, sometimes at the expense of family time and group needs. By encouraging involvement in activities outside the home, middle-class parents position their children to receive more than an education in how to play soccer, baseball, or piano. These [children] acquire skills and dispositions that help them navigate the institutional world. They learn to think of themselves as special and as entitled to receive certain kinds of services from adults. They also acquire a valuable set of white-collar work skills, including how to set priorities, manage an itinerary, shake hands with strangers, and work on a team.[4]

Lareau contrasts this approach, which she terms "concerted cultivation," with the "natural growth" practices more common among lower-income parents: "The limited economic resources available to working-class and poor families make getting children fed, clothed, sheltered, and transported time-consuming, arduous labor. Parents tend to direct their efforts toward keeping children safe, enforcing discipline, and, when they deem it necessary, regulating their behavior in specific areas. . . . Thus, whereas middle-class children often are treated as a project to be developed, working-class and poor children are given boundaries for their behavior and then allowed to grow."[5]

Neither of these approaches is inherently better for children: poor and working-class children, for example, experience more freedom in their play, and, unlike their heavily supervised middle-class counterparts, they must learn to work out disputes with their peers without adult intervention. But the particular skills and dispositions—the *cultural capital*—that middle-class children develop are the ones most valued by educators, and so these children enter school with a built-in set of advantages. That sense of "fit" can, in turn, impact students' enjoyment of school. Paul Willis found that working-class students' experiences of marginality and disadvantage in school fostered feelings of resentment or rebellion against schooling; instead of offering a chance at upward mobility, school became the reason why "working class kids get working class jobs."[6] Beyond schooling, class-conditioned habits may also help middle-class job seekers gain access to favorable positions. Michèle Lamont, speaking of white-collar workplaces, explains that "managers favor employees who resemble them culturally, and . . . corporate success partly depends on making other managers 'comfortable' by conforming in cultural matters and not 'standing out.'"[7] How, then, do parents prepare their children for success in this arena?

The children of mothers in my study were not yet joining sports teams, taking piano lessons, or learning to interact with authority figures. They were, in most cases, years away from entering grade school. Instead, the skills they were learning tended to be more basic: how to chew solid food or use a toilet; in a few cases, they had yet to be born! Given the class differences I have described during the previous chapters, how might differences in mothers' reproductive body projects, as well as their likelihood of treating body-care practices as a source of identity and agency, impact children's own bodies and class dynamics?

## Moderation, Cosmopolitanism, and Informed Consumption: Middle- and Upper-Class Values

As described in previous chapters, middle- and upper-class mothers frequently voiced strong health and body-care values that they tied to their identities; their ability to articulate and follow through on a diet or birth plan expressed their rigid agency. Thus, it comes as no surprise that these women had some very clear ideas about what food, health, and activity-related values they wanted to instill in their children. Such was the case for thirty-two-year-old Stephanie Brewer, a white mother of two living in California:

> It was important to me that my children eat people food, grown-up food, because I'm not willing to make four different meals. If my husband and I want to eat salmon and brown rice and sautéed bok choy, then that's what the kids are getting. . . . The other thing was that I wanted my kids to be raised in a way that included them in the kitchen, because I love to cook. So it's great to get my kids' feedback about what they want for dinner. Earlier in the week, I said, "Okay, Olive, we have to have either chicken or pork with our dinner. Which one do you want?" And she said chicken. I said, "Okay, well what's a vegetable that you want to have with it?" She said sweet potatoes. Well, I thought, my husband's favorite is my chicken and sweet potato curry: "Olive, can I make a curry with some spice?" And she said, "I don't like spice." So I said, "Okay, if I make it not spicy will you try it? It has the chicken and the sweet potatoes." And sure enough, she ate it! I heaped yogurt into it to cut the heat. Boy, I was so proud of her! And my son, who's been a little picky towards meat, he even ate it. . . . Good god, my kids eat curry! These are things I can pat myself on the back about, because I've worked really hard to get them to the point where they're even willing to try it. And that we can sit as a family and enjoy it.

Stephanie's pride in her children's expansive palates—and in her own work to develop their tastes—was evident throughout our conversation.

She rattled off a list of other challenging foods her kids liked and noted that she'd even begun a blog dedicated to the topic of feeding young children and developing their appetites, which she shared with friends and acquaintances. And while Stephanie enjoyed the fruits of her labors on an everyday basis, passing on her love of food to her children, she was particularly thrilled to show off Olive's cosmopolitan tastes when their family traveled abroad:

> When we were in Tuscany, we ate Tuscan food, and my daughter ate everything that was put in front of her. That's the part of Italy that my family is from, so it was food that was extremely familiar to Olive because it's the flavors and things she's already aware of. She blew away a couple that were tourists that were four seats away from us, that she ate a mound of pasta with clams and pesto and all sorts of things in it. And they were like, "How can you get your three-year-old to eat that stuff?" And I'm like, "I don't know—it's 'cause she's eaten it before." . . . It's really fun. And it makes us want to take our kids to go travel. We took my daughter to Ireland when she was fifteen months old, and we didn't know really what to expect with traveling with a toddler. I was nervous about feeding her, because at that point I was still very specifically managing what she ate. I hadn't said, "Okay, let's just feed her whatever." So we tried it, we just fed her whatever we were eating. And we discovered that she has a love for chicken liver pâté. So we would order chicken liver pâté at least once a day, and she would just eat her little crostini with pâté. She also discovered a taste for Guinness, which was probably not so good! [laughing] It's always bad when your fifteen-month-old is like "Ahh!" after the pint glass! But that's fine—it's everything in moderation.

Three main themes stand out from Stephanie's account of teaching her children how to eat. First, Stephanie endowed food and the rituals surrounding it (family dinners, planning and cooking a meal, sampling local cuisines while traveling) with a great deal of personal importance, citing both cultural heritage and the traditions of big family dinners that she and her husband grew up with. Sharing these rituals with her children involved work and active cultivation, but also joy. Second, food symbolizes the *lifestyle* to which Stephanie wanted to habituate her children. Stephanie was not worried about affording nutritious food or making cheap food palatable; instead, she encouraged her children to request and negotiate for diverse foods, including some that were fairly expensive ("Around the holidays we always have Dungeness crab. My daughter was fighting people for the last claw. That's awesome!"). Likewise, Stephanie assumed that international vacations would be an ongoing part of her children's future lifestyles, and she was proud that they were already starting to consume food in ways that marked them to others as sophisticated, adventurous, and cosmopolitan. Third, wrapped up in these efforts at cultivating children's tastes is the implicit message that food is abundant and resources are limitless; concerns about food waste or getting adequate nutrition are noticeably absent.

The theme of teaching children to become knowledgeable and discerning consumers was widespread among middle- and upper-class mothers. These women modeled learning about and controlling what they put in their bodies, and, like Stephanie, they helped children practice that kind of decision making for themselves. Engaging in these practices, however, required a significant investment of time. Mixed-class mother Kirsten Cooper (white, thirty-eight, LH) linked the ethical consumption of "real foods" to her identity, explaining, "I want [my daughter] to see where the food comes from. I think that's honest. I think it's easy to forget what this [food] is and where it came from, and how you get it. So squishing some apples in the juicer and making juice every once in a while is super important. It is who we are from a philosophical standpoint." Later, Kirsten described taking her children to a farm to watch cows being milked, repeating her belief that knowing about food's origins matters because "it makes up who we are." Yet, despite Kirsten's breezy comment about squishing some apples in a juicer "every once in a while," she and other women who engaged in these types of practices—mostly middle- and upper-class mothers, though Kirsten herself was mixed-class—devoted significant amounts of time to consuming in this way. Hillary Kirk (white, twenty-six, HH) explained, "It's very important to me to try to prepare whole foods, rather than prepackaged foods. I like to control the ingredients that I put into things. I spend a lot of time reading recipes and looking for different ideas." For Hillary and her peers, the ability to control exactly what she was putting into her own body and that of her children made the time investment worthwhile. And Diane Sperry (white, thirty-seven, HH) exclaimed to me about how proud she was to have concocted a recipe for homemade black bean brownies "instead of opening up a package of Oreos and tossing those at [the children]." Of course, the convenience and shelf life of packaged foods like Oreos, generally made possible by artificial preservatives, made them particularly appealing to poor families on a budget who could not afford food spoilage. But for the high-status women I spoke to, avoiding such foods was more than a form of economic distinction: it was a lesson in appropriately middle- and upper-class modes of consumption, offering a blueprint for children's own future body projects.

Bree Turner (white, thirty-three, HH) spoke about what she hoped these lessons could mean for her children's personal development more generally, explaining,

> I want [my kids] . . . to have good information about the choices they make, whether it's nutrition or drugs and alcohol or media or friends, whatever it is. And I want them to feel secure enough in themselves to be able to make decisions that feel good for them. I want them to be confident, secure, and curious. I want them to know how to find answers. In terms of nutrition, I want them to understand why I'm asking them to eat vegetables, maybe why I steer them away from sugar. . . . I guess, teaching them how to find answers themselves, too.

Essentially, Bree hoped to empower her children by equipping them with a process for making decisions about their bodies; she did not assume that she could predict the answers, but she believed she could help them ask the right questions and develop the self-confidence to follow through on whatever they chose to do. And while Bree acknowledged that, at some point, her children would be making their own decisions about what to eat, she hoped to model the kind of balance that she, herself, valued: "It's life. Enjoy it, you know? Especially when you have kids. You don't want to shut out everything that is fun for them, because when they get to a point when they can make their own decisions, they may not make the right decisions. We eat pizza. We eat ice cream and all that fun stuff, too. [Laughing] Sometimes you do better than others, and you just have to accept it." Anya Novak (white, forty, HH) agreed that "moderation is a better approach" than either the strict healthism her parents had pursued when she was a child or the junk-food habit she developed in response when she went away to boarding school as a teenager. She hoped that her son would eat in ways that supported his body's development, but she explained that these habits were about more than just his physical body: "For myself, it symbolizes more than just physical nourishment. It has to do with self-care, an idea of, like, 'It is my job to take care of myself.' That's part of what being alive is about—self-nourishment. And that doesn't mean just food. It could mean exercise and doing your job and making money and saving money. You know, all of the things that we would do in an ideal sense to take care of ourselves. So I think food is a symbolic thing. It's real in and of itself, and it also symbolizes more than that." For Anya, as for Bree and other middle- and upper-class mothers, teaching their children to make good, thoughtful decisions about food was both practical (for well-being) and symbolic of becoming the "right" kind of person: informed, deliberative, and responsible. Few of the middle- and upper-class mothers I interviewed spoke explicitly about trying to transmit advantages to their children through their bodies. A handful of women across classes described maternal body projects like breastfeeding or taking fish oil supplements intended to boost children's brain development. Mothers typically framed these and similar practices as "giving children the best possible start in life." Such framing gestured toward the status work women were performing but did not specify the particular competitive advantages they hoped their investments would produce. More commonly, middle- and upper-class mothers spoke about wanting their children to have a healthy relationship with food, to make informed choices about their bodies, and to feel a sense of ease, freedom, and moderation—rather than anxiety and constraint—when making those choices.

## Cleanliness, Clear Rules, and Averting Ill Health: Poor and Working-Class Priorities

Like middle- and upper-class mothers, poor and working-class women typically did not frame their hopes for their children's bodies in terms of class, mobility, or conferring advantages. Yet the specific goals and priorities these two groups outlined to me looked quite different. Where class-privileged women aimed to endow their children with sophisticated, cosmopolitan tastes, poor and working-class mothers spoke about helping their children appear tidy and clean. Where the former emphasized the importance of teaching their children skills for critical thinking and informed consumption in health, the latter embraced simple, clear rules about "good" and "bad" foods. And while middle- and upper-class women spoke about finding a balance between indulgences and more healthful choices that would enable children to develop positive attitudes toward food and their bodies, poor and working-class women spoke about family health histories dotted with chronic illnesses like diabetes and their fervent hope to break the cycle with their children.

## Cleanliness

For many poor and working-class women, the challenges of keeping young children clean and presentable loomed large. May Campbell (forty, LL), a Black Caribbean immigrant living in Florida, told me she prioritized teaching her children "how to wash their private areas real good! I make sure I watch them when they're taking a shower, especially my daughter. She likes to . . . wash real quick. [I tell her] 'Go in there and take your time, girl!'" I asked May why this was important to her, and she answered, "There are some people that I've met, oh my goodness! I think, 'Can't you smell yourself coming out of your house?'" May's disgust was palpable, compounded by her belief that the odor came from someone's genitals. To be a person who went out in public smelling so bad—or to be the mother of such a person—would be a source of deep shame.

Other low-income mothers shared May's focus on teaching good hygiene to their children. Several were anxious about avoiding cavities and ensuring their children had good teeth. Grace Kellogg (white, twenty, LL), meanwhile, described cleanliness as an important competency for adult life—and for boys like her son, especially. She explained, "He's going to have to learn how to do his own laundry, just to make him self-sufficient. He'll learn how to take a bath, and he'll learn how to take a shower, comb his hair, and brush his teeth. . . . Teaching him how to cook his own food so he can eat healthy, because I think a lot of boys just don't know how to cook, so they buy McDonald's. I think boys are more unhealthy than women." For Grace, raising a boy into a young man who could care for his own bodily needs—rather than depending on his mother or girlfriend to perform that labor—was a particularly important value, even though her son was less than a year old when I spoke to her. And in the lessons that Grace, May, and others imparted to their children, we see an emphasis on self-reliance, rather than the consumerism more common in middle- and upper-class parenting.

Projects like May's and Grace's are complicated by social inequality. On one hand, all children, regardless of background, need to learn basic hygiene: how to wash their hands, brush their teeth, clean properly after toileting, and more. Virtually all children get messy and, from time to time, resist caregivers' best efforts to tidy them up—my own child, for example, has been known to scream bloody murder when I try to wipe jam off her face. On the other hand, the moral and material *stakes* of children's cleanliness are tangled up with race, ethnicity, and class. Throughout US history, people of color, immigrants, and low-income groups have long been symbolically linked to dirt and disease. Grime and body odor may sometimes represent actual material inequalities, such as when a child goes to school wearing unwashed clothes because they lack laundry facilities at home and cannot afford the laundromat. At other times, nonwhite and immigrant individuals may get labeled as smelly (due to the foods they eat or the grooming products they use) or unkempt (especially if their hair deviates from European style norms) as a result of observers' racist and xenophobic attitudes. The costs of being labeled as such are significant: even in the twenty-first century, Black women with natural (unstraightened) hairstyles still face employment discrimination for looking "unprofessional." And parents who are judged by the state as failing to properly groom, clothe, or feed their children risk being charged with neglect and losing custody; poor and working-class families are especially vulnerable to such accusations due to their more frequent contact with state agencies. Under these circumstances, low-income mothers' emphasis on tidiness and respectability takes on added significance: they are not only maintaining children's physical bodies but also safeguarding their children's dignity and well-being in a way that white and class-privileged parents must rarely consider.[8]

## Clear Rules

Poor and working-class mothers' health and body-care lessons to their children also highlighted a shared emphasis on simple, easy-to-remember rules for distinguishing "good" foods from "bad." Whereas many middle- and upper-class mothers valued informed consumption, deliberating over the nutritional and environmental impact of their eating choices and encouraging their children to do the same, poor and working-class mothers sought to impart clear-cut health rules to their children: salad, vegetables, water, and exercise were good; sedentary lifestyles and sugary or greasy "junk" foods were bad.

Shawna Blanchard (Black, twenty, LL) laughed as she told me, "I really want my daughter to be healthy, like be involved in sports and eat good. She shouldn't have my eating habits at all!" India Brown (Black, twenty, LL) concurred: "I'm trying to teach her to eat right. Eat the good things and not the things that Mommy eats, all the sweets and chocolate." And Janie Reed (Black, twenty-one, LL), who was pregnant with her first child, anticipated facing a similar struggle: "It's hard to eat less sweets and greasy food. . . . I eat the foods on the WIC checks and feel good about that. I don't exercise too much, though. . . . I'd want my daughter not to make my mistakes of eating fast food. She should eat home-cooked food, or, like, at a steak house or Chinese. She should exercise, if she wants to." For young women like Shawna, India, and Janie, envisioning healthy values for their children meant breaking with the eating habits and tastes that they, themselves, had grown up with. Gaby Romero (Latina, twenty-nine, LL) believed that she needed to force herself to eat salads for her son's sake. She explained, "Even stuff that I eat [but] I don't like, I want him to eat them. I need to teach him how to eat them." And Tina Smith (Black, forty-one, LL) laid out her food priorities in clear terms: "I try to eat healthy. I try to eat fruit every day, and a glass of water, stay away from junk, try to set an example for my son."

In interview after interview, I was struck by low-income mothers' near-identical mental maps of "good" and "bad" foods. To be sure, there were patterns in the ways middle- and upper-class mothers assigned value to particular foods and health practices ("real" versus processed foods, homemade versus store bought, organic versus conventional agriculture), but none was so uniform as the value systems that lower-income mothers held and attempted to follow. Three explanations seem likely. First, virtually all of the low-income women I spoke to were enrolled in WIC, a federal nutrition program that puts a high premium on nutrition education. Federal and state guidelines determined which foods WIC would subsidize, as well as the content of the pamphlets and learning aids that WIC staff used in their nutrition classes and one-on-one counseling sessions. It is unsurprising, then, that a group of women enrolled in a standardized education program would come to share a set of fairly standard ideas about health and nutrition. Second, the psychological impact of poverty makes these guidelines' simplicity particularly attractive. Researchers have found that conditions like food and housing insecurity force people to expend mental resources strategizing how to make ends meet, which imposes a "cognitive tax" on the mental energy they have left for making decisions.[9] Thus, while women in comfortable financial circumstances sought to develop children's deliberative and critical thinking skills when it came to making health-related choices, women with fewer resources valued having a streamlined decision-making process and aimed to pass this on to their children; the benefit of these schemas of "good" and "bad" foods was that they offered a way to make good-enough choices for health and then move on, reserving mental energy for the more pressing problems and decisions children would face in their lives.

Third, though, the role of class here appears to be cultural as well as material. Whereas women with low incomes *and* low educations typically viewed WIC's simple food rules with appreciation, mixed-class mothers from higher-class backgrounds and levels of education looked askance at those rules. College-educated Gita Potter (Asian, twenty-seven, HL) explained to me that WIC's nutrition counseling sessions felt redundant to her, saying, "I know we're kind of starving students, but I like to prepare healthy things anyway and have balanced meals just because I know that's better for our bodies. I can see how if I wasn't raised in a household where those things were taught that this might be really groundbreaking news. But it's really pretty simple stuff that I know about." Although she had to adapt the healthy meals she planned to her family's limited budget, Gita still placed a premium on informed consumption and balance similar to what most high-status mothers did, suggesting that the *cultural value* of consuming in this way was more important to her than whatever mental load she might ease by follow-ing a "simple" set of rules. Annie Castro (white, twenty-nine, HL) also received WIC aid but framed her relationship to it as a taxpayer, not a client: "I'm very thrilled that they're so strict about how things have to be whole grains, very limited processed stuff. I like knowing that my tax dollars are going toward making children healthy. A lot of people don't have good nutritional practices—especially, I feel, a lot of people who use these types of programs. . . . Even if people don't have healthy lifestyles then it will hopefully help with child obesity, make sure they can't neces-sarily repeat what they experienced as kids or in their family." Thus, for highly educated, mixed-class women like Annie and Gita, "simple" rules and restrictions were for other types of WIC clients—people who grew up in households where they were not taught to eat well and for whom even basic categories of "good" and "bad" food might be "groundbreak-ing news." Mixed-class women were well aware of the class connotations of their health habits, and they took pains both to symbolically distance themselves from poor mothers and to ensure that their own children would grow up with a more nuanced, high-class understanding of health and nutrition. Thus, the preference for simple, straightforward health guidelines among low-income, low-education women would appear to be the product of both economic and class cultural influences.

## Averting Ill Health

The last major theme in low-income mothers' accounts of their hopes for children's bodies was avoiding specific health problems. People on the lowest rungs of the socioeconomic ladder have significantly higher risks of chronic illnesses like asthma, diabetes, and hypertension, the result of a complicated set of factors including chronic stress, malnutrition, physically taxing manual labor, exposure to pollution/environmental racism, inadequate preventive healthcare, and more. Those problems are most pronounced for racial/ethnic minorities, especially African Ameri-cans.[10] For many of the poor and working-class women I spoke to, then, protecting children from the health problems common in their families was a major priority.

Lynne O'Brien (white, twenty-seven, LL) outlined the hopes she had for her children's futures, explaining, "Well, I want them to take care of their self. I want them to get up every morning, brush their teeth good. I want them to eat healthy, don't eat junk. Don't get me wrong, I do it, I'm guilty. . . . I don't want that for them because then they're going to start doing it all the time, and then they're going to start being like me: out of shape, out of energy, feeling tired all the time." Lynne acknowledged that teaching her children to do things differently would represent a big change from how she was raised: "My dad gave us pizza whenever we wanted it. We could eat junk food all day long if we wanted to. . . . I want my kids to know that they can't have cheeseburgers or pizza all the time. It's the grease that bothers me, because when I got pregnant with [my daughter], I ended up getting gestational diabetes. It's not something I want them to have to go through, and I already know that I'm going to end up with full-blown diabetes because my parents have it, my sisters have it." Nicole Johnson (Black, twenty-two, LL) cited a similar family history to Lynne's, and a similar determination to break the cycle:

> We do have high diabetes in our family, they actually thought my brother was going to have diabetes when he was little. . . . Sugar is very, very important [to avoid]. We drink Crystal Light, which is pretty good. We let the sugar still sit in the cabinet. If it was at my mom's house, it would be gone [because it got eaten]. I don't want to have diabetes; I'm next in line since I am the oldest in my generation bracket. I want to try and break it, and then it's supposed to be able to skip a generation. So hopefully it skips two, since I don't want my daughter to have it.

Stories like Lynne's and Nicole's, encompassing family histories of diabetes as well as heart disease, chronic obstructive pulmonary disease (COPD), and other diseases linked to diet and lifestyle, were common among my low-income respondents. When I asked these women about their own relationships with their bodies and what they hoped to give their children, they shared some of the same concerns about body image and preventing substance abuse that middle- and upper-class women cited. But where, for class-privileged women, drugs and eating disorders represented some of the biggest bodily threats their children might face, for poor and working-class women it was the risk of disability and premature death from illness that weighed most heavily on their minds. Whether as a result of inherited genetics or inherited family health habits, many of my respondents believed they and their children were predestined to struggle with the same bodily challenges that their own parents and grandparents had lived with—and died of.

Vanessa Garfield (white, twenty-five, LL) put these fears most clearly when she laid out her reasons for monitoring her children's diets:

> We don't get a lot of junk food or anything like that. And for their teeth too. We try not to give them any sweet drinks. They just drink juices, because I want them to be healthy. And they're hyper enough without any sweets! . . . My dad loved junk food. He had a heart attack at thirty-five and they tried to get him to stop eating so much junk food and so much fast food, but he just didn't do it. So now we see on my dad's side of the family a lot of obesity because of it. I don't want my kids learning the same thing.

As Vanessa saw it, even suffering a heart attack at age thirty-five did not convince her father to adopt healthier eating habits—his love of fast food was too powerful. He eventually died after he had a second heart attack. Vanessa believed the only way to protect her children from a similar fate was to shape their dietary tastes and habits from an early age, keeping them from ever developing the love of "junk food" that she believed killed her father. She avoided sugary sodas and made a point of offering vegetables to her children at every meal, though getting them to eat the vegetables remained challenging.

In summary, poor and working-class mothers shared clear priorities for their children's health and well-being that were shaped by the class-related material and cultural conditions of their everyday lives. The women I spoke to did not frame their choices and goals as tied to class, but the daily risks and stressors they described were a far cry from the lifestyles that class-privileged women discussed. In a society that frequently stereotypes poor and other marginalized people as dirty, mothers in my study sought to ensure children's dignity by making sure they always looked tidy and presentable. In a context where people facing job or housing insecurity experience the constant mental drain of juggling bills and other obligations, low-income mothers sought to give their children simple, clear-cut guidelines for healthy living to reduce stress and facilitate good decision making. And, growing up in families where premature death and disability from chronic illness was a common oc-currence, mothers I interviewed were fiercely determined to break the cycle and help their children live relatively pain- and disease-free lives.

## Cultivating Classy Bodies: Mixed-Class Mothers' Conscious Transmission of Embodied Advantage

Privileged mothers frequently told stories about teaching their children to become informed consumers, though these women rarely named these lessons' connection to social status. Yet, a small number of women described making intentional choices to pass on advantages through their body-care practices to their children's bodies. Beyond the general statement many women gave about trying to give children the best start in life, a handful—predominantly mixed-class women—were more explicit about what they were trying to accomplish, and how. Lee Mendoza (white, thirty, HL) named these dynamics when she explained her decision to breastfeed: "In my heart, I honestly believe that breast milk is better for brain development. . . . I'm the first person ever to graduate college [in my family]. My husband is the first person from his family to graduate college, and between us we have five degrees, so [education] is very important to us. And I know that breastmilk—and I think studies back this up—leads to better brain development." For Lee, whose upward mobility—and her husband's—had been hard won, ensuring her child's ability to succeed in school was of the utmost importance. Breastmilk, she believed, was the key to that success. Kirsten Cooper (white, thirty-eight, LH) likewise drew connections between her efforts to cultivate her child's body and his ability to succeed in school. She imagined consumption choices and activities that would benefit him: "I think sports are really good for a person to develop intellectually. . . . Especially team sports, it gives you something that other academics can't, that help you in academics and other parts of life." Kirsten's focus on the developmental benefits of sports echoes the *concerted cultivation* practices that Annette Lareau describes in her sample of elementary-aged middle-class children and their parents: children were primed for success not only through learning to read or do math but also through a set of mutually reinforcing, carefully mapped out academic and extra-curricular activities.[11]

Meanwhile, graduate student Juana Reyes (Latina, twenty-nine, HL) focused on the cognitive benefits she could accrue for her child through prenatal exercise and linked those to potential social benefits later in life: "I was reading a lot about exercising and being pregnant, and how . . . kids tend to have a better IQ, better self-esteem about themselves, and tend to be more athletic, like wanting to go play outside and be on sports teams and whatnot." Alongside these practical advantages, she spoke more generally about balance and body image in ways that mirrored middle- and upper-class mothers' answers, while also seeking to break with the habits she had learned in her own, working-class childhood:

> I don't want [my son] to have a negative relationship with food. I want him to make healthy choices, but at the same time every now and then having ice cream, or if we go out and he wants to get a Slurpee, I think that's okay. Definitely not every Friday, like I did when I was growing up! I want him to know that food is available and that we nourish our bodies with food, so I don't want him to grow up worried about "Oh, I'm too fat" or "I don't look as good as the other boys do."

Like most other mixed-class women in my study, Juana's explanation of how she wanted to raise her son blended higher- and lower-class patterns of response (cultivating a positive body image and relationship to food; breaking "bad" habits inherited from one's family of origin). An important marker of Juana's upward mobility was that, while she did want to make sure he didn't worry about the availability of food— something more common among low-income families—her most pressing worry was to protect him against feeling that "I don't look as good as the other boys."

The trend of mixed-class women talking about transmitting class advantages to their children in explicit terms is noteworthy. As previous chapters have discussed, mixed-class women are more likely than most to have mixed social contacts, drawing support and wisdom from peers and family members in a range of social statuses. At times, these mixed contacts can cause women to hold a mixture of beliefs and practices reflecting higher- and lower-class patterns; much of the time, though, mixed-class women's ideals for health and body care most closely resemble those of women who share their *educational* level, thus providing evidence for the strong influence of class culture—knowledge and norms, not material wealth—on the contents of women's reproductive body projects.

Mixed-class women are also more likely to experience status anxiety and to invest time and energy in drawing clear boundaries between themselves and lower-status women who are, for one reason or another, still too close for comfort. Many of these mothers had only recently achieved upward mobility, and they knew their toehold in the middle class was tenuous. Those who had experienced downward mobility— usually women with college degrees who had become eligible for WIC— sought to reassure me and others that this status was only temporary, the result of conscious choices (graduate school, becoming a stay-at-home parent) that would bolster the family's long-term social or financial well-being. For such women, framing their work on children's bodies as intentional status cultivation was strategic, one more way to position themselves as properly middle class, even as they lacked material resources to fully enact that performance. Their *awareness* of those efforts as linked to class was a product of their social position: with one foot in each world, they had the clearest view of the class patterns in health and body-care practices that solidly higher- or lower-class women performed without a second thought.

## Conclusion

Middle- and upper-class women worked on their children's bodies in several ways, endowing their children with expansive consumer tastes, skills for critical thinking and informed consumption of health information, and bodily attitudes that balanced moderation with pleasure. While these women did not, typically, frame these projects as status reproduction, such was the effect of their efforts. Furthermore, mothers' *performance* of investing in their children's bodies also bolstered their own status as subjects with the right, high-status values. Poor and working-class women offered a different set of lessons to their children: they emphasized good grooming and the importance of a tidy appearance; they followed simple, time-saving rules about "good" and "bad" categories of food; and they strove to protect their children against the myriad chronic illnesses and life-shortening conditions that were widespread in their communities. While these lessons offered practical solutions to the material and social circumstances of low-income families' lives, they also may have marked LL women as being out of step with higher-status food and body-care trends in the eyes of their healthcare providers or other audiences.

Mixed-class mothers were the exception in my study. Unlike most women, several of them explicitly described the efforts they put into cultivating their children's bodies as human capital investments; they believed that the skills, tastes, and habits they taught their children would provide a competitive advantage in children's schooling and careers. In short, they consciously framed their caregiving as *status work*. Such was rarely the case for higher- and lower-status mothers. When low-income mothers with high school degrees taught their children that sugar was "bad," they saw this as doing all they could to give children the best start in life: providing clear, easy-to-follow rules that could help children avoid tooth decay, unwanted weight gain, or even chronic illness. When college-educated women with high household incomes taught their children to make informed choices about their diets and to cultivate expansive palates, they, too, believed they were doing all they could to give their children the best start in life: helping kids develop healthy, balanced attitudes about food and body image while preparing them to make travel and cross-cultural fluency part of their lifestyles. In nearly all cases, higher- and lower-status mothers did not identify these lessons as imparting class-connected knowledges and competencies. Does that mean they were not performing status work?

I would argue that they were still engaging in status work, albeit unconsciously. Through the specific information, health habits, and values that mothers sought to instill in their children, two sets of class-differentiated priorities emerged. First, middle- and upper-class mothers spoke highly about the importance of moderation and a balanced attitude toward food and other pleasures; they did not want their children to eat or drink to excess, but neither did they want kids to develop disordered or obsessive relationships to diet and exercise. Second, mothers in this group urged their children to explore their different options—for food, healthcare, or anything else—and to make well-researched, informed decisions. They imparted this lesson both by modeling it (talking to children about their own body-care choices, showing them where different foods came from) and, as Stephanie Brewer did, by engaging children in a give-and-take dialogue about how to cook or consume a meal. Third, class-privileged women focused on preparing their children to take part in the social rituals of eating, whether sampling local cuisines when traveling or sitting down to a family meal. These priorities reflect the particular circumstances of middle- and upper-class lifestyles: having the financial freedom to consume exciting and high-quality foods, the mental energy to develop personalized body-care regimens, and the time and means to travel.

Poor and working-class mothers converged on a different set of health and body-care priorities for their children. First, they aimed to make sure their children were clean and well groomed and, when children were old enough, prepared to take responsibility for their own health and hygiene. Second, mothers in this group shared a fairly uniform set of rules for "good" and "bad" health habits: vegetables, salads, home-cooked foods, and fruits were "good," as was living an active lifestyle; sugary and greasy foods, as well as smoking and other drugs, were "bad." Mothers in this group varied in the extent to which they felt capable of following these rules themselves—some strove hard to model the right habits for their children, while others adopted a "do as I say, not as I do" approach—but virtually all believed that following these rules would lead to better health for their children. Third, they focused on the personal benefits to children's health that could result from these practices. Given the high prevalence of chronic illnesses, disability, and early death in low-income mothers' families and communities, they spoke less about the abstract good of, say, supporting environmentally sound farming than about the more immediate good of helping their children live long lives free of pain and illness. As with middle- and upper-class mothers, low-income women's priorities developed in response to their social and material context.

Clearly, the differences in mothers' lessons to their children about body-care practices and priorities *result from* class differences in resources, social norms, and everyday lifestyles. But can these classed habits and knowledges also *contribute to* class differences in the future? To use the language of Paul Willis and social reproduction theory, do bodies help ensure that "working class kids get working class lives" or middle-class kids get middle-class lives?[12] My data—drawn from a single point in these children's early lives—do not, on their own, allow me to answer that question. But the scholarly literature on status and social reproduction suggests that these bodily tastes and habits can indeed carry status consequences in later life.

The class-specific forms of cultural capital that children learn growing up are best suited to helping them thrive within their families and communities of origin. The concept of *habitus*, developed by Pierre Bourdieu, holds that different social strata nurture and reward different cultural knowledges and habits: where one class habitus might prioritize toughness, self-sufficiency, and a preference for deeds over words, another might instead place a premium on sensitivity, collaboration, and communication.[13] Each set of attributes and competencies has its own uses; what enables middle- and upper-class people to retain social power and prestige is their ability to ensure that major social institutions— especially schools—will recognize *their* preferred forms of cultural capital as the *right ones* (for educational success, professionalism, and so forth). Annette Lareau's 2003 book, *Unequal Childhoods*, documents the extent to which early childhood socialization and family resources can set children up for success or struggle in school: middle-class children experienced school's norms and rules as being in harmony with the interactional styles they learned at home; poor and working-class children, on the other hand, felt a strong sense of dissonance between the two settings and encountered teachers who interpreted their interactional styles as inattentive or disruptive. Beyond schooling, studies have found that hiring managers tend to seek out workers who match their idea of a "good" employee: generally, someone much like themselves who comes from the same habitus, attended the same type of school, and/or who can be vouched for through a shared social acquaintance.[14] Not surprisingly, such patterns can reproduce not just class hierarchies but gender and racial inequalities as well.

Thus, while lower- and higher-status women did not invest in their children's human capital with the same intentionality as mixed-class mothers, they nevertheless habituated their children into developing class-appropriate forms of cultural capital. The question is, Do these bodily forms of cultural capital—the health- and body-specific knowledges, tastes, and habits that cluster together among people of a particular social status—translate into socioeconomic advantage or disadvantage? Put another way, how might the divergent bodily attitudes and practices that mothers in my study nurtured in their children set them up for later life struggles or success?

Past research shows that schools offer informal rewards to students who have the right kinds of bodies, or who use their bodies in the right ways. Patrick Brady found that peers and teachers alike placed athletes at the top of a high school's social hierarchy.[15] Students described athletes as "good" and "important" to school spirit and institutional identity; meanwhile, they perceived that teachers gave preferential treatment and individual attention to athletes while excusing them from some of the behavioral policing that other students were subjected to. These modes of favoritism can help athletic students feel that school is a place where they fit in and are valued, not to mention insulating them from punishments that might derail their academic careers. C. J. Pascoe's study of masculinity among American high school boys likewise illustrates the high social status of middle-class, athletic, good-looking boys (and the relatively marginal positions of boys who were effeminate, working-class, or had "bad" skin or teeth).[16] Similarly, high school girls whose bodies fall outside of dominant standards for heterosexual femininity—slender, fit, wearing stylish clothes, and attracting attention from high-status boys—face social marginalization, bullying, and harassment from their peers.[17] These hierarchies of popularity and belonging, while not perfectly correlated with academic and later life success, certainly create an environment where some students—physically fit, conventionally attractive, nondisabled, heterosexual—receive more resources, support, and validation in school than others.

Beyond high school, bodies continue to matter for social and professional success. Christian S. Crandall found that parents of fatter-than-average daughters were less likely to offer those daughters financial support for college, independent of parents' ability to pay and children's academic prowess (sons did not face a financial penalty for being fat).[18] Scholarships and preferential college admissions policies for athletes, meanwhile, privilege students who have developed their bodies' abilities to an impressive degree. Contrary to popular belief, however, these scholarships are not a primary pathway for lifting low-income students into the middle class: the students most likely to benefit from these policies are the middle-to-upper-class children of parents with college degrees.[19] Such students have received both the lesson that athleticism matters and the resources to afford equipment, coaching, travel to competitions, and more.

Once young people enter the workplace, bodily inequalities continue to shape decisions in hiring, promotion, mentorship, and more. Previous research has found persistent income disadvantages among fat employees;[20] in various professions like law and academia, people who are perceived as conventionally attractive are more likely to receive positive evaluations and be hired into more prestigious positions.[21] Kristen Barber notes that white-collar, professional men increasingly consume luxury grooming services like manicures and scissor haircuts to get "superior, more 'stylish' hair, separating them from 'grease monkey' mechanics at the barbershop whom they believe don't care—and don't need to care—about how they look."[22] And Ryan Westwood, an entrepreneur writing for *Forbes*, argues that businesses should "hire athletes," both because of the cooperative skills and work ethic that athletes supposedly cultivate and because "it works to a company's advantage to hire health-minded people who take care of themselves."[23] Notably, Westwood's *Forbes* article is just one in a long line of similar pieces that the business magazine has published about the benefits of hiring athletes, often while advertising networking services that cater specifically to current and former college athletes.[24] Clearly, the fit, athletic body—along with the personal virtues it is taken to represent—is held in high regard in corporate America.

Some of the bodily attributes that schools and workplaces value may be due to the luck of the genetic draw, but many are the product of the different kinds of work that people put into managing their body's shape and appearance. It is not only what you are born with, but what you do with it: the body as achieved status. The tastes and resources people bring to those projects are, as this chapter has described, shaped by class. As Carl Stempel finds, "Dominant class adults use participation in sports to draw boundaries by strenuously working on their bodies to produce disciplined, high performing and achieving selves. Engaging in strenuous sports is a practical, embodied way to maintain distance from the classes who are lazy 'couch potatoes' that 'let themselves go.'"[25] Put another way, high-status people use their bodies and the specific work they do on them—often through strenuous aerobic exercise like training for marathons and triathlons or through trendy branded fitness programs like CrossFit and Peloton—to demonstrate their moral character: health focused, but also determined, competitive, and ambitious. In this way, they distance themselves from the working class, prove their fitness for managerial and professional careers, and develop bodies that look and act the part for those careers. Employers take these bodies' appearances as evidence of an applicant's intangible qualities like drive and commitment, as well as their ability to fit in to workplace culture.

Many of the highly educated, middle- and upper-class mothers in my study held athleticism and bodily self-control as central pillars of their own self-identities. In the lessons they taught their children—to make informed decisions about health, to develop cosmopolitan consumer tastes, and to cultivate a sense of moderation in their exercise and consumption habits—these women were reproducing those same ideals in the next generation. But while high-status mothers' body-care lessons were calibrated to helping their children gain or retain socioeconomic advantage, poor and working-class women's efforts instead aimed to insulate children against the dangers of poverty, particularly as it intersected with racial inequality. These women hoped to prevent their children from developing chronic illness, especially through the transmission of simple, easy-to-follow rules for healthy eating; and they hoped, too, to protect children from being stigmatized as dirty, unkempt, and low-class. WIC guidelines reinforced low-income women's approaches, protecting their children against the worst risks of poverty, but not instilling the sort of bodily cultural capital that would facilitate their movement into the middle class, either. In this way, mothers in my study all did their best to care for and develop their children's bodies and body-care habits while simultaneously—and, largely, unconsciously—reproducing a two-track system of bodily habits and values. The outcome of this status work, to paraphrase Paul Willis, is how working-class kids get working-class bodies.

# Conclusion

## Healthism as a Function of Class

Pregnancy, childbirth, and the postpartum period entail rapid changes in the feel and function of mothers' bodies. These changes are simultaneously biological, representing the interplay of genes, hormones, and physiology, and social, reflecting the medical, economic, and cultural circumstances in which reproduction happens. Meanwhile, the women in my study recounted stories about the individual efforts they undertook to help ensure that things went right with their pregnancies or to give their child the best start in life. From these stories there emerged clear patterns of class differences in how women dealt with their bodies during and after pregnancy. These differences, I suggest, offer us a window onto broader class differences in how inequality is embodied in the contemporary United States.

Middle- and upper-class (HH) mothers spoke eloquently about the reproductive body projects they had taken on. They nurtured horizontal, give-and-take relationships with peers and medical providers that would help them develop their expertise in body-related matters; they offered coherent narratives of their body-care choices that affirmed their values and identities as health-conscious mothers; and they approached the unpredictable events of maternal embodiment with a determinedly rigid agency, striving to maintain or regain control of their bodies when things did not go according to plan. In all of these ways and more, HH mothers' orientations to health and body care aligned with normative healthist ideologies. Women in this group pursued their reproductive body projects with near-religious devotion, investing significant time, resources, and emotional energy into the pursuit—and they taught their children to do the same.

In contrast, poor and working-class (LL) mothers offered accounts of their health and body-care practices that were ambivalent at best.

These women, especially those who were in their teens or early twenties when they became parents, sought support and advice through vertical, hierarchical relationships with medical experts or older women like their own mothers. They tended to resist crafting elaborate narratives of their body-care values, instead either conceding that they believed their choices were not ideal or redirecting the conversation to an area—such as career aspirations—that they felt better represented their identity. And when faced with the bodily changes and surprises of maternal embodiment, LL mothers were less likely to reassert rigid control than to react flexibly, accepting that some things were out of their control. To be clear, LL women cared about their health. And they especially cared about their children's health. But they did not adopt health as a spiritual quest: they did not embrace healthism. For mothers in this group, pursuing health was pragmatic, a priority only insofar as they could obtain concrete benefits for themselves or their children. These women focused on practical, straightforward measures they could adopt to improve their well-being, and they resisted the demand that they sink endless time and resources into their reproductive body projects. This view, likewise, shaped the body-care lessons they taught their children.

## Class Cultures and the Pursuit of Bodily Distinction

What accounts for these differences? At the start of this book, I posited three possible explanations for class differences in body-care habits: (1) economic inequalities, particularly in access to health products and services; (2) disparities in health literacy and information; and (3) class cultural or ideological differences in the use of the body to demonstrate distinction. Mixed-class mothers, it turns out, help us understand the roles played by each of these factors.

### Financial Freedom or Constraint

In the kinds of reproductive body projects they took on, their tastes in consumption, and their degree of investment in healthism, mixed-class mothers most closely resembled HH or LL women who shared their level of education. In other words, highly educated mothers receiving WIC aid (HL) resembled wealthier, college-educated women

(HH) in terms of the ways they talked about their health and bodies and in the priorities they outlined to me. Financial constraints sometimes limited their ability to consume in the ways that they desired: Noura described her fantasy of owning a top-of-the-line Ergobaby infant carrier, and Christine explained that fresh produce felt like a luxury "because it seems expensive and immediately perishable, so you have to move through it kind of fast." Still, these women adopted many of the same practices and values as wealthier women with similar levels of education. If their budgets were to increase, they would know exactly how and where to spend the money to consume in recognizably "classy" ways.

In contrast, mixed-class women from working-class backgrounds and/or who had not completed college (LH) typically had the financial means but not the habits to gather and consume health knowledge and services in middle-class ways. They felt uncertain when participating in healthist conversations with middle-class peers, describing feelings of being excluded or else, like Cass, adopting a receptive stance in which they listened to other mothers without engaging in the give-and-take of body-care tips more typical of HH women's friendships. These patterns all suggest that current household income is not the main determinant of women's reproductive body projects.

## Health Literacy and Information

Another possible explanation of class differences in body-care practices is health information and literacy.[1] It stands to reason that college-educated mothers—who had similar patterns of behavior regardless of financial status—might have greater knowledge or research skills that could help them navigate the conflicting health messages that new mothers receive. Mixed-class women like Annie and Gita described the lessons they received at WIC—reminders about the health benefits of breastfeeding, diagrams illustrating portion sizes or the nutritional content of different foods, and more—as "simple" or "basic." When Annie's WIC counselor urged her not to drink sugary sodas, Annie replied with disgust, "Yeah, we don't do that." Mixed-class Nicki Lindsay, describing a breastfeeding roundtable discussion she took part in at WIC, likewise framed her difference from LL "girls" thus:

Some of the girls were not as interested, and I was kind of trying to encourage that breastfeeding is a good thing, and that it doesn't hurt after a
while. That you get used to it, and it's so convenient. But I feel like [WIC]
could have done a better job at encouraging them in that. It's tough,
because the poor nutritionist feels like she's speaking to a wall, and the
people are kind of looking at her like, "I don't really want to talk." . . . But
I thought it was good. I thought that some of the girls that were in there
maybe came away with a different mindset, and maybe would consider
breastfeeding, when maybe they wouldn't before that.

For mixed-class mothers like Nicki and Annie, the problem of poor
and working-class women's "unhealthful" practices came down to a lack
of education and information. WIC, they believed, could help remedy
that problem. Poor and working-class (LL) women in WIC, however,
did not always see things this way. Working-class mother Tina Smith defended her decision not to breastfeed as a matter of choice, not ignorance:
"I guess they figured you don't have the information so they kind of push
it [breastfeeding] on you. No, it's not that. It's a choice that I've made."

These competing accounts capture some of the tension inherent in
the health-literacy explanation of class differences in body-care practices. On one hand, WIC does provide information about nutrition and
other body-care practices, and many enrolled women, especially young
mothers, voiced appreciation for that information. Even though Gita
and other mixed-class mothers called that information "basic," it nevertheless ensured a foundational level of knowledge about scientific and
medical guidance for maternal embodiment in low-income women. On
the other hand, class-differentiated body-care practices and preferences
persist. When asked whether her choice to use formula was based in ignorance of the benefits of breastfeeding, Tina replied, "No, it's not that."
Thus, class disparities in health information do not fully explain the
class-differentiated patterns in health and body-care behaviors, either.

## Bodily Distinction

Neither economic nor health literacy frameworks can fully explain class
differences in health-related behaviors. Those differences, however,
serve a signaling function: for someone attuned to these differences,

even subconsciously, observing how a person consumes "health" trends can offer strong evidence of that person's class of origin. Reproductive body projects are a performance, and audiences interpret that performance to make determinations about the individual's social and moral status. Most mothers did not explicitly cite status as their motivation for engaging in various body-care and consumption practices—they usually named health and well-being as their goals—but these classed patterns persisted nonetheless.

Mixed-class mothers—both HL and LH—were the exception to this rule. Of all the women I interviewed, mixed-class women were the most likely to explicitly link their body-care practices to social status. For these women, who sometimes found themselves in uncomfortably close proximity to lower-status women (and who did not want to be mistaken as low-status themselves), caring for and presenting the body in recognizably middle-class ways served as a means to draw clear symbolic boundaries, a way of saying, "I may be poor, but I'm not like those *other* women in the WIC office." As the case of these mixed-class women makes clear, the body and its care function, for new and expectant mothers, as a site for performing cultural distinction. These women's stories also help us understand the roles played by economic inequalities, access to information, and the interplay between individual choices and structural forces.

## Public Policy (Mis)Understandings of Classed Health Behaviors

At play here are not massive differences in health information but, rather, class-differentiated choices about what to do with that information: middle- and upper-class (HH) women, as well as highly educated mixed-class women (HL), prioritized gathering and acting on as much health information as they could get. Reflecting their class cultural devotion to healthism, these women tended to be early adopters of new fads in diet and fitness, to self-identify as "Type A" or "researchers," and to tie their identities to their body projects. Poor and working-class (LL) mothers tended, instead, to take an à la carte approach to health and body-care practices, picking and choosing the ones that best fit their families' needs. These women were more likely to place health and body optimization on a back burner relative to other household priorities, and they also were less likely to despair if they did not attain some particular goal they had set for their bodies.

Perhaps sensing this lack of enthusiasm for healthism among poor and working-class women, the Champions for Change, an initiative of the California Department of Health Services, launched a public information campaign in 2010 designed to foster the "right" health attitudes. Entitled "Hero Moms," this campaign created billboards and "Hero Mom Success Cards" featuring images of real moms—mostly women of color—and slogans to promote healthier choices. As I boarded the bus to visit a WIC office or walked to a coffee shop for one of my interviews, I passed billboards with messages like these:

"My Budget, My Rules. Rule #6: Eat Right When Money's Tight" (billboard, CA Champions for Change)

"My Shopping Cart, My Rules. Rule #5: Buy More Fruits and Vegetables" (billboard, CA Champions for Change)

"I find the time to make healthy meals." (Hero Mom Success Card #6)

The campaign offered free tips for eating healthy on a budget or saving time, suggesting, for example, that women might cook large batches of food to save on meal-prep time later in the week. The campaign's decision to focus on time and financial barriers was appropriate: lack of time and money were indeed two of the biggest challenges LL women cited when explaining why they did not follow all of WIC's health guidelines. But what the Champions for Change campaign suggested as a remedy was, essentially, to do more with less—to pursue individual, behavioral solutions to the structural problems of poverty and the social determinants of health.

Viewed in light of the stories low-income mothers told me, these money-saving tips appear cruelly ironic. They urged mothers to budget for fresh fruits and vegetables, yet many women I interviewed pointed out that perishable produce was an unaffordable extravagance during lean times, and even the Champions for Change materials acknowledged that children might need to be exposed to a new food six or more times before they began to like it.[2] In other words, prioritizing fresh produce meant, for many people, risking significant food waste. Meanwhile, the suggestion that cooking and shopping in bulk can save time is true, but only for people who have a lump sum of money to acquire food in bulk, adequate kitchen facilities in which to prepare it, and the space (and reliable refrigeration) to store it safely once it is cooked.[3]

There are a couple of problems with the approaches the Champions for Change campaign pursued. This campaign fell into the common trap of proposing individual, behavioral solutions to deep, structural inequities. Further, to the extent that class differences in health behaviors exist, any attempt to change those behaviors requires understanding the *structural drivers* of individual behavior, rather than chalking them up to a lack of information or will power. While these instances of misrecognition are sampled from the Champions for Change campaign, they are emblematic of the fundamental misunderstandings that many public health interventions—including WIC and other programs—espouse when attempting to improve maternal and infant health in low-income communities.[4] It is precisely these types of misunderstandings that *The Reproduction of Inequality* seeks to correct.

## Individual Solutions to Structural Problems

One problem with the campaign's messages was that they implied that individual behaviors are the primary driver of health disparities across racial and socioeconomic groups. Some individual health behaviors do matter quite a lot—for example, smoking during pregnancy poses a significant, proven risk of harm to a developing fetus as well as to the smoker. But on the whole, health behaviors are *intermediary determinants* of health, layered on top of an underlying foundation of social, structural determinants of population health: stratification due to race, class, gender, and more; the material conditions in which people live and work; the social networks and resources to which they have access; and the whole range of social policies that mediate people's access to affordable housing, education, healthcare, and other resources.[5] When it came to the health and body-care habits of low-income mothers, the Champions for Change campaign offered similar solutions to those espoused by the WIC program and by mixed-class women. Essentially, these slogans framed low-income women as lacking adequate information or correct health priorities, and offered free tips and education—as opposed to material aid in the form of free or low-cost food, housing, and medical care—as the solution. In this way, they individualized the problem of systemic health and body-care disparities.[6]

### Misrecognizing the Effects of Ascribed Status as an Achieved Virtue: Taste and Choice as Consequences of Class

The Champions for Change campaign also attempted to treat the *symptoms* of class and racial/ethnic differences in health behaviors rather than their *root causes*, arguably a more serious error in the campaign and one that ignores the structural factors mothers face. My interviews with low-income mothers suggest that poverty, specifically, impacts behavior. But as evidence from low-income, mixed-class mothers shows, that impact is a bit more complicated than simply having or lacking the ability to afford things. Instead, the effects of poverty on behavior are mediated by culture, appearing as questions of *taste* or *choice*.

First, building on Bourdieu's concept of class bodies, different groups develop different class-conditioned tastes and habits: what Bourdieu calls the "taste of luxury" and the "taste of necessity."[7] Simply put, people develop a taste for consuming those things they can afford, particularly early in life. Even if they experience class mobility as adults, they are likely to retain preferences for the sorts of foods and other experiences they were exposed to as children. Thus, mothers' choices about food and consumption were not driven solely by affordability; they were also driven by class-conditioned bodily tastes. In practice, this meant that many poor and working-class women I spoke to had difficulty using the nutritious free foods they received through WIC; they disliked the low-fat milk or whole-grain bread that their vouchers specified, and so they either struggled to consume foods that were distasteful to them or, in some cases, shared the food with another household member who did not mind the flavor.

Second, stress and poverty drastically limit the amount of cognitive energy people have for worrying about their health. Anandi Mani and her colleagues have found that "being poor means coping not just with a shortfall of money, but also with a concurrent shortfall of cognitive resources."[8] When people are dealing with financial insecurity and juggling competing needs, financial strategizing takes precedence. The result is often a decreased capacity to plan or fully think through other, less urgent matters. This sort of cognitive load certainly showed up in poor and working-class mothers' narratives. Women spoke to me about the exhaustion they felt, both mental and physical, when trying to navigate health advice, keep track of appointments with doctors and public-assistance programs, and care for their young children on limited budgets. They described the stress of living in large, extended-family households to pool resources and get help with childcare, and they noted the physical and emotional pain of having to return to work soon after childbirth because they could not afford to take their full allotment of unpaid maternity leave (if they were even lucky enough to qualify for unpaid leave). When Champions for Change offered these women advice about how to budget or make calculated, rational decisions for their families, it was missing the point. The problem was not that poor and working-class women were doing too little thinking about the consequences of their choices, health-related or otherwise; it was that they were doing too much. Instructing these women to make better choices, without relieving some of the cognitive load they bear as a result of their financial circumstances, is unlikely to yield a significant change in behavior.

In summary, public health policy and programs like the Champions for Change campaign treat class and racial/ethnic health disparities as a result of individual health behaviors, rather than structural factors. And in their efforts to change disadvantaged women's health behaviors, they fail to understand the material underpinnings of those behaviors, viewing them instead as a function of individual values, knowledge, and will power. Any serious attempt to improve public health across classes needs to reevaluate these simplistic beliefs.

## Solutions, Part I: Making Poor and Working-Class Women More Like Middle-Class Women

From the perspective of health outcomes alone—whether we measure maternal and infant mortality rates, rates of chronic illness, or longevity—middle- and upper-class people do better. Policies that seek to remedy these inequalities are typically trying to make poor and working-class people more like middle- and upper-class people in their health behaviors and outcomes. Fortunately, several of these challenges share a solution: reducing poverty and inequality. When more members of a population have access to education, income, healthcare, and other social resources, maternal and infant mortality rates decline.[9] At the individual level, Mani and her colleagues found that the decreased cognitive capacity of their impoverished research subjects was not fixed from a young age; when subjects were retested after they became more economically stable, their ability to reason showed marked improvement.[10] If policy makers like those behind the Champions for Change campaign want to enable low-income women to behave more like middle- and upper-class women in regard to their health and bodies, the solution is not cheap, but it is simple: give them access to the kinds of resources that middle- and upper-class women have.

Some of this help could be targeted during the maternal embodiment period. Public-assistance programs like WIC could increase their monthly allowances for food and streamline the processes for enrolling and for booking or rescheduling an appointment; they could even allow clients to renew benefits remotely, thereby freeing up clients' time and mental energy for work or childcare. Medicaid could expand its coverage options for pregnant and postpartum clients to give them greater choice in medical providers and in the settings where they give birth. Birth attendants known as doulas, whose role is to support the laboring person, could be funded and trained specifically to advocate for disadvantaged clients who may not know how—or that they have the right—to request different care options for their birth.[11] And if government health agencies like the Centers for Disease Control are serious about encouraging more women to breastfeed, they should push for federal mandates for employers to provide *paid* parental leave so that postpartum and lactating parents are not forced to choose between their health and breastfeeding relationship on the one hand and having enough money to support their families, on the other.

More broadly, getting poor and working-class women to focus more of their energy on making healthful decisions requires reducing inequality across the life course, not just during the short window of pregnancy and the postpartum period that constitutes maternal embodiment. Low-income mothers I interviewed typically wanted to take better care of themselves, but struggled to find the time. These women told me about the unpredictable work schedules of their minimum-wage jobs that made pumping and maintaining their milk production nearly impossible; they told me about the challenges of getting to the grocery store and doctors' appointments when their car was broken down and they had to wait for a friend to give them a ride; and they told me how, when money was tight, they saved the most nutritious food for their children and made do with granola bars for themselves. Until these pressures are relieved, poor and working-class women will never have the material resources or cognitive capacity to focus on "health" in the same way that their middle-class peers do. In short, the solution to the health deficits of low-income households (both real and imagined) is not simply to give them advice about how to do more with less; it is helping them achieve enough financial stability that they can do more by having more.

## Solutions, Part II: Making Middle-Class Women Less Like Middle-Class Women

Should middle- and upper-class mothers act as our yardstick for measuring optimal health and body-care practices and attitudes, though? The deficit model assumes so, holding that class-privileged women's practices are ideal, and that poor and working-class women's practices can be explained by what they lack. Certainly, there are many features of middle- and upper-class motherhood—the ability to afford high-quality childcare; flexible hours and maternity-leave benefits; and a sense of ease when navigating healthcare settings and requesting personalized care, to name a few—that all mothers could benefit from. But the stories middle- and upper-class women shared with me about the costs of keeping up with healthism should give us pause. In this final section, I invite readers to think beyond the deficit model to ask, What changes might we hope to see in how even middle- and upper-class women approach health and body care in the future? If "health" is both a matter of bodily well-being and a status marker, are there any down sides to the middle- and upper-class preoccupation with living health-focused lives?

### Wellness Work and Gender Inequality

Most middle- and upper-class women in my study reported taking on disproportionate responsibility for family health and wellness labor relative to their husbands. They conducted the bulk of the research on child nutrition and development questions; crafted plans for managing bodily transitions like potty training or introducing new foods; and acted as conduits for body-care information received from children's teachers, healthcare providers, and other peers and professionals. When these women professed a commitment to egalitarian parenting, they often had to perform the additional labor of presenting their research to their partners so that they could make decisions as a couple. Previous historical and sociological scholarship on mothering in the United States shows how cultural expectations for "good mothering" have expanded over time: even as devices like laundry machines and vacuums have decreased women's household labor in one area, cultural expectations for women's investment of time and energy in their children have increased.[12] The demands that women engage in what Sharon Hays calls "intensive mothering" and what Annette Lareau calls "concerted cultivation"—time-intensive, intentional investments in children's intellectual, social, and physical development—are particularly pronounced for white, class-privileged mothers.[13] Black women, in contrast, are more likely to prioritize paid work and financial provision as key to good motherhood.[14]

These same gender and racial dynamics showed up when it came to women's particular responsibility for household wellness and body-care labor. Middle- and upper-class women in my study, most of whom were white, were already a pretty physically healthy group, as were their children; they also were more likely to be presumed healthy by healthcare providers and other audiences. Yet their healthist commitment to optimizing their bodies' tastes and capabilities expanded to fill all of their available time. Mothers who left full-time work to care for their children poured the same level of time and energy into developing their body-care expertise that they had once devoted to their careers. They described writing blogs about child nutrition, inventing recipes to entice their children to try new foods, and devoting hours to Internet searches so that they could make informed choices about vaccination or ask their child's pediatrician for specialized help.

The marginal benefits to many of these health and body-care practices seem slight compared with the labor they take to accomplish: Diane Sperry's homemade black bean brownies were probably more nutritious than a package of Oreos, but was the difference truly worth the time it took her to make them? More to the point, how many hours in a week or a year did white, class-privileged women like Diane devote to these kinds of projects relative to their husbands? Past studies have shown that race/ethnicity, more than class, affects the size of the gender gap in household labor among heterosexual couples. But cross-racial differences in the division of household labor seem to be due almost entirely to the amount of time women spend on household labor; men's participation does not vary much across racial groups.[15] If healthism demands that poor and working-class families—who are disproportionately people of color—devote more time and energy to the pursuit of various body projects, that time and energy would most likely be extracted from women, thereby increasing the gender gap in their households' labor. For this reason, we should be cautious about the unintended gender consequences of pushing low-income families to adopt middle-class patterns of investment in "health" and body care: pursuing healthism in middle-class ways could increase gender inequality within households.

## The Personal Toll of Healthism

Devoting time to nutrition and body-care habits can, of course, bring rewards beyond "health" or status. Learning to bake our own bread, sharing and exploring diverse food traditions with our friends and families, or testing our bodies' limits through exercise can all be meaningful, pleasurable experiences. But there is a difference between body projects taken on for one's own satisfaction and those taken on out a sense of obligation or fear. For too many of the middle- and upper-class women in my study, the expectation that they intensively focus on health and bodies was not a source of joy but, rather, a site for distress and anxiety.

Lara Noble, describing her struggles with bulimia, expressed this distress most clearly: "I hated the mental jail . . . of spending 90 percent of my waking hours thinking about food, weight, calories, exercise." Michelle Carter described how, as a teenager, she "tried to be bulimic" to get the sort of body she felt she ought to have, but "I couldn't do it. It was horrible and I hated myself and I hated to throw up." Diane Sperry added, "I try to avoid the mirror. I don't like the shape of my face, the shape of my nose, and the paleness of everything." Long before becoming mothers, middle- and upper-class women had internalized restrictive social norms for how their bodies should look. Trying to achieve that look often became a harmful preoccupation, as evidenced by the large numbers of women who admitted to past or current eating disorders, and it left many women feeling shame or hatred toward their bodies.

When it came to the care of their children's bodies, too, many women in this group expressed deep feelings of inadequacy. Misty Clifford, describing her efforts to eat right during pregnancy, recounted, "It was difficult, because sometimes my body cooperated and craved what I needed. I craved good things like fruit. But sometimes I felt like I needed to eat more protein and the thought of protein disgusted me, and I couldn't eat it. And then you get so tired, and I'd think 'Oh! I could really use a cup of coffee right now.' I found that mom-guilt set in really early." Misty elaborated on "mom guilt" at length, describing how every choice she made for her child was laden with worries about whether she was doing the right thing. In her pregnancy eating habits, she tried to listen to what her body was craving, but she still felt bad that she was not craving the "right" foods. Suzanne Walsh, meanwhile, did not want to admit to some of her friends that she received Pitocin and epidural anesthesia during childbirth. Her husband bragged to their friends that her childbirth was "natural," because the epidural had worn off when the time came for Suzanne to push, and Suzanne hesitated to correct him. That class cultural pressure did not end once the baby had arrived, either. Suzanne continued, "[Breastfeeding] is like the culture of natural childbirth. Amidst the upper middle class that I'm in, it's assumed people will breastfeed. And I think that, especially in this area, there is judgment against people who don't breastfeed. One of my good friends' partners couldn't breastfeed and they had to give formula, and I know she felt bad about that. She felt ashamed." Women who invested heavily in healthism also suffered heavily when their bodies failed to meet the high standards to which they were held. Even though women like Suzanne and Misty made their choices in light of their bodies' needs—Misty tried to eat intuitively based on what she was craving, Suzanne accepted pain medication to ride out the excruciating back labor caused by her baby's positioning—they still felt, somehow, that they had failed to make the healthiest choices.

In short, external and internalized healthist pressures to think about and perfect the body caused many middle- and upper-class women to feel guilt, shame, and self-hatred. While some women found enjoyment in these pursuits, the pressure to get everything right made even fun hobbies like home cooking feel, too often, like a competition and an obligation. I would argue that, faced with these normalizing judgments, women from low-status backgrounds, like mixed-class Dani Hahn, tended to have the more emotionally well-adjusted responses: "If I can't handle it, I'm not going to be mad at myself."

## Maternal Embodiment as a Harbinger of Future Resilience

When women like Dani—mostly poor or working-class—responded with *flexible agency* to the bodily changes of pregnancy and the postpartum period, they were demonstrating a mindset that could benefit them later in life. Middle- and upper-class mothers, as we have seen, espoused *rigid agency* in their efforts to control their bodies. They set strict goals for their maternal bodies, such as breastfeeding for a year or having an unmedicated birth, and took steps to achieve those goals. Losing control felt like a crisis. Some women successfully wrested back control by pushing themselves harder or spending additional time and money to resolve bodily problems; others struggled to accept their loss of control and experienced distress as a result. Many described their experiences of early motherhood using words like "traumatic," and turned to therapy to help them move on.

The rigid agency most common among class-privileged women refuses to acknowledge the truth that bodies change. Fortunately for these women, most (though not all) of the bodily changes specific to pregnancy, childbirth, and lactation are transient; most (though not all) people will return to their pre-pregnancy state of being able to tie their own shoes, wear pants without elastic waistbands, eat and exercise as they wish, sneeze without leaking urine, and so on. Thus, some middle- and upper-class women were able to weather these changes by compartmentalizing. As Charlotte Moran put it, "The feeling after I had my baby of wanting to get back to a pre-baby body is totally about regaining control of this body that I feel I've lost control of." Essentially, for Charlotte, the bodily loss of control that pregnancy entailed was bearable only because she conceived of it as temporary.

Not all bodily changes we experience throughout our lifetimes will be temporary, though. As feminist disability scholar Rosemarie Garland-

Thomson reminds us, "Disability is the most human of experiences, touching every family and—if we live long enough—touching us all."[16] For many of the young, fairly healthy women I interviewed, pregnancy represented their first real brush with impairment, their first experience of living in bodies that did not feel or function as they were accustomed to. Poor and working-class women's *flexible agency* left them better equipped to roll with those changes, suggesting that they may have better resilience for facing the more permanent changes in bodies and abilities that come with aging and impairment.

## Healthism and the Reproduction of Inequality

Lastly, one of the central contentions of this book has been that reproductive body projects and the status work mothers do as they care for and nourish their children's development are a site for displaying and reproducing social-status inequalities. In the contemporary United States, healthism—similar to educational attainment—helps legitimate social inequalities, disguising privilege as merit. Many of the expensive and time-consuming "health" practices that high-status people pursue as part of their everyday lives offer only marginal or unproven benefits to well-being; such practices do, however, help individuals display moral and status distinction and signal their cultural fit to schools and employers alike.

Ironically, those status distinctions help to perpetuate the very socioeconomic inequalities that drive actual health disparities in the United States.[17] One response, then, might be to bridge the divide between lower- and upper-status people's lifestyles and practices. The deficit model assumes that the solution is to increase the amount of time and money that low-income mothers spend on "health," to compel them to do more. What if, however, we asked middle- and upper-class women to do less? Spend less time focusing on their own body projects (except to the extent that these body projects are actually enjoyable or address a known health issue), and spend less time micromanaging children's bodies and development? What if we rethought the moral value of endless investment in "health"?

This would be a difficult thing to ask. Despite how miserable the pursuit of "health" made many of my class-privileged respondents, they also believed it was their moral duty and a way to express love for their children. Neoliberal parenting norms teach us that loving our children means investing everything we can in them, giving them every competitive advantage we can muster (even if we also believe in the principle of equality of opportunity, at least in the abstract). As long as the performance of "health" and various high-prestige body-care practices carry status benefits, asking middle- and upper-class women to do less means asking them to give up some of their privilege, or at least to pass on slightly less privilege to their children.

Perhaps, however, it would be helpful to think of this change less as denying children an advantage than as gifting them with distance from the food and body obsessions that so many adults carry, freeing them from the consuming focus on the body that Lara Noble termed "mental jail." Previous research has found that being in the presence of "fat talk"—disparaging remarks about a person's body size or dietary habits, including one's own—can increase a person's risk of developing eating-disordered patterns of thinking or behavior.[18] The authors of that study suggested that interventions in friendship groups, where peers agreed to work on eliminating fat talk from their conversations, could help to reduce those risks. In the context of the current project, perhaps middle- and upper-class women who find themselves in peer groups where "health talk" is common could adopt a similar approach. By dialing down the frequency with which they compared reproductive body projects, these women might experience a corresponding reduction in the level of competitiveness and insecurity they felt in these interactions. At the same time, poor and working-class women less fluent in healthist discourse might find fewer social barriers to conversing with middle- and upper-class peers.

## Looking to the Future

In the introduction, I posited that maternal bodies are a microcosm of larger social trends involving the body as a site for displaying and reproducing inequality. What conclusions might we draw, then, for bodies in society more generally?

Most obviously, everyone, regardless of social status, deserves respectful, responsive healthcare that supports them in making choices for their own bodies. People who are marginalized on the basis of race, ethnicity, class, sexuality, gender, and more face hurdles not only in accessing care but also—once they have found a provider—in having their concerns and preferences taken seriously. High-quality health and body care should be a right, not a privilege.

But, while high-status people come to expect responsive care from their providers—as they should—they also mistakenly expect that they will always be able to control their bodies, shaping their bodies' form and function to their will. The flexibility that poor and working-class mothers in my study were forced to learn due to the constraints within which they operated could also serve them well over the life course as their bodies inevitably do change; there are lessons, here, about the resilience that can come from accepting that our bodies will not be young, healthy, and nondisabled forever.

For me, one of the most personally meaningful takeaways from these mothers' stories is the knowledge that babies come into this world and are fed, clothed, and cared for in all manner of ways and grow up just fine. The intensive focus on optimizing "health" is not a universal or timeless norm but, rather, a fairly recent and culturally specific one. The accounts of immigrant women—who took a more measured approach to US health norms because of their exposure to multiple cultures—and low-income women, especially Black women, who resisted the pressure to define themselves by their health practices, are especially instructive here. Future research on these women, as well as on some groups not included in the current study—middle- and upper-class Black women, for example, and LGBTQ+ parents—could help to further illuminate the interplay of class, race/ethnicity, and gender in different groups' approaches to caring for their own bodies and those of their children. The more we are exposed to a wide range of body-care practices and philosophies, the less pressure we will likely feel to adhere to one model.

Speaking of that model, what if we treated the pursuit of health less like a religion to which we must profess our devotion and more like a hobby? To be sure, some attention to our bodies and health is necessary to live and have an acceptable quality of life. But the same could be said of preparing food or keeping our homes clean: it is true that you must eat or you will die, and that you must maintain your living space and clothes or risk hazards like mold, electrical fires, and so on. But not everyone who feeds themselves aspires to cook gourmet meals, and not everyone who keeps their home clean is interested in getting featured in lifestyle magazines. So, too, might we think about health and body projects: some attention to health and fitness is ideal for maintaining a decent quality of life, but pursuits beyond that are more a reflection of personal enjoyment or taste—a chosen hobby—than they are strictly necessary. The benefits of this shift could be twofold: at the individual level, perhaps more of us could learn to love and enjoy our bodies (rather than viewing them as a source of guilt, shame, or punishment). At the societal level, perhaps we could begin to let go of the notion that class-conditioned bodily tastes and habits mark some people as better—smarter, more disciplined, more cultured—than others. In letting go of healthism, we might reduce social inequality, and in the process improve the health of our society.

# ACKNOWLEDGMENTS

Writing this book, whose long gestation has spanned multiple jobs and cross-country moves—not to mention the gestation and birth of my own child—has been made possible by the material, emotional, and intellectual support of an amazing group of people.

I am grateful for the financial support I received while conducting and writing about this research, including a grant from the UC–Berkeley Center for Race and Gender and Miami University's Wiepking Distinguished Visiting Professorship. At Wheaton College, a Wheaton Research Partnership Grant brought me the chance to work with a student research assistant, Kayla Sifre, on compiling and recoding interview transcripts.

I owe particular gratitude to the intellectual communities that nurtured my exploration of these topics. At UC–Berkeley, members of the Department of Women's and Gender Studies such as Barrie Thorne, Charis Thompson, and Minoo Moallem challenged me to expand my intellectual horizons beyond the disciplinary boundaries of sociology. In the Sociology Department, I received critical engagement and advice from Irene Bloemraad, Vicki Bonnell, Michael Burawoy, Mike Hout, Kristin Luker, Sandra Smith, and Loïc Wacquant. These scholars offered me sage advice, critical engagement, and unfailingly high standards.

Members of the Berkeley Sociology of Gender Working Group, including Jessica Cobb, Freeden Oeur, and Jennifer Randles, were some of my earliest critics and cheerleaders as I began mapping out the research that would set me on the path toward writing this book.

Raka Ray served as my dissertation chair, but that title feels inadequate to describe the breadth of her mentorship and the powerful and multiple ways in which she modeled feminist scholarship and molded her students into a lasting intellectual community. Raka organized her students into a writing group that met regularly to discuss everything from the challenges of research and writing to professional development as we waded into the academic job market. Abigail Andrews, Kemi Balogun, Jenny Carlson, Dawn Dow, Katie Hasson, Kimberly Hoang, Kate Maich, Jordanna Matlon, Sarah Anne Minkin, and Nazanin Shahrokni—the members of "Team Raka"—gave generously and untiringly in their feedback, reading and commenting on multiple drafts of my work. Writing can be an isolating experience, but as a part of this group, I never once felt that I was doing it alone. Without their support, I would not have been able to write this book.

I owe particular thanks to Kimberly Hoang and Heidy Sarabia, who met with me weekly by phone while we were each conducting fieldwork. Heidy and Kimberly offered feedback on my first, tentative efforts at writing about my findings, reading so carefully that they knew my data almost as well as I did. Jenny Carlson challenged me to engage more deeply with theory in my work; in long discussions held over coffee or cocktails, she urged me to tackle difficult theoretical concepts head on and to believe that I had something worthwhile to say in response. Dawn Dow, meanwhile, became my writing accountability partner and coauthor; much of what I know about writing a book came from watching her do it first.

Thanks, also, to colleagues who advised and offered feedback on this project once I turned to revision: Anita Mannur, Natalie Boero, Hyun Kim, Karen McCormack, Justin Schupp, Sabrina Speights, and Javier Treviño.

This book would not have been possible without the enthusiastic participation of the seventy women whose interviews form the core of this book. These women welcomed me into their homes, used precious childcare hours to speak with me, demonstrated their diapering and infant-feeding techniques, and shared intimate details of the many emotional and physiological challenges they faced in becoming mothers. I joke sometimes that interviewing parents about their kids is easy, because they usually have a lot to say. But the truth is, these women were incredibly patient with me, a twenty-something who had spent very little time around babies and who had never even heard of attachment parenting. Thanks, also, to the Women, Infants, and Children staff members in California and Florida who ushered me into the WIC office and took the time to answer my questions about their work in the program.

I owe a special debt of gratitude to my mother, Ginny McDaniel, who went above and beyond the call of familial duty. Not only did she house and feed me during one stretch of fieldwork but also, having recently completed her own graduate thesis, she offered to transcribe many of my completed interviews. During early morning walks, we reflected together on some of the more striking comments that cropped up in those interviews, and she frequently left me notes in the transcripts' margins comparing subjects' stories to her own experiences as a parent.

A special thanks to Ilene Kalish and her colleagues at NYU Press: Mary Beth Jarrad, Yasemin Torfilli, Alexia Traganas, Emily Wright, and many others. Ilene offered me encouragement and grace when, in the final stages of writing and revising the manuscript, I encountered two major disruptions: first, the birth of my child, and second, the COVID-19 pandemic. Through it all, Ilene kept faith with me and helped me find a home for my manuscript with series editor Jennifer Reich. Jennifer's feedback, informed by her own research on parents' health choices for their kids, helped me strike a balance between empathy and critical distance in my writing.

Finishing a book under these circumstances was possible only with the help of a team of family and paid childcare providers. At Fort Hill, Tori, Martha, Kris, Kelly, Ashley, Mark, and Jo, along with the rest of the staff, nurtured our child's growth while working overtime to keep her safe in the midst of a pandemic; when everything shut down, Ben Sambrook joined our bubble and became a source of dependable and loving care. And as soon as they were able, three sets of amazing grandparents—Ginny and Doug, Hilary and Rick, Marty and Kath—stepped in to help out, too.

Finally, I dedicate this book to my brilliant spouse, Jen Malkowski, and to our bold, inquisitive child, Jamie. While Jen has supported me in untold ways since the start of this project, they played a key role in helping me finish it: on more than one occasion, they ordered me out of the house for a solo writing retreat, shouldering all the parenting and other household duties so that I could write without distraction. An accomplished author in their own right, Jen understood what I needed without my having to ask. I hope to have written something they will enjoy reading! Jamie, you bring me unimaginable joy. Thank you for sharing my time with this project; I hope, in some small way, that I have become a better parent because of it.

# APPENDIX

## *List of Interview Subjects*

TABLE A.1. High-Education, High-Income Mothers

| Pseudonym | Age | Age at 1st Child | Race | State | Number of Children | Marital Status | 2011 Income Quintile | Class * |
|---|---|---|---|---|---|---|---|---|
| Alison Correia | 29 | 27 | White | FL | 1 | Married | 4 | HH |
| Amanda Katz | 30 | 28 | White | FL | 1 | Married | 4 | HH |
| Amy Chen | 35 | 31 | Asian | CA | 2 | Married | 5 | HH |
| Anya Novak | 40 | 38 | White | CA | 1 | Married | 5 | HH |
| Bree Turner | 33 | 30 | White | CA | 2 | Married | 5 | HH |
| Britta Larson | 39 | 39 | White | CA | 1 | Married | 4 | HH |
| Charlotte Moran | 32 | 31 | Biracial (Asian, white) | CA | 1 | Married | 3 | HH |
| Diane Sperry | 37 | 28 | White | FL | 2 | Married | 4 | HH |
| Emily Fischer | 31 | 31 | White | FL | 1 | Married | 5 | HH |
| Fiona Garcia | 39 | 37 | White | CA | 2 | Married | 4 | HH |
| Greta Davies | 40 | 38 | White | CA | 2 | Married | 5 | HH |
| Hillary Kirk | 26 | 26 | White | FL | 1 | Married | 3 | HH |
| Jen Vargas | 29 | 28 | Biracial (Latina, white) | CA | 1 | Married | 4 | HH |
| Jessie Wozniak | 31 | 29 | White | FL | 1 | Married | 4 | HH |
| Joan Zimmerman | 38 | 33 | White | FL | 2 | Married | 4 | HH |
| Kimberly Peters | 30 | 27 | White | FL | 3 | Married | 4 | HH |
| Lara Noble | 40 | 37 | White | CA | 2 | Married | 5 | HH |
| Lori Kent | 29 | 29 | White | FL | 1 | Married | 4 | HH |
| Lucy Wolff | 33 | 33 | White | FL | 0 | Married | 4 | HH |
| MacKenzie Gervais | 30 | 27 | White | FL | 1 | Married | 4 | HH |
| Masha Begovic | 34 | 31 | White | FL | 3 | Married | 4 | HH |
| Michelle Carter | 29 | 27 | White | FL | 2 | Married | 4 | HH |
| Miranda Hughes | 36 | 34 | White | FL | 1 | Married | 5 | HH |
| Misty Clifford | 31 | 29 | White | CA | 1 | Married | 5 | HH |
| Nadia Bernard | 36 | 35 | White | CA | 1 | Married | 4 | HH |
| Rhea Weston | 23 | 22 | White | FL | 1 | Married | 5 | HH |
| Sonia Gallo | 35 | 31 | Latina | FL | 3 | Married | 5 | HH |
| Stephanie Brewer | 32 | 28 | White | CA | 2 | Married | 5 | HH |
| Suzanne Walsh | 35 | 34 | White | CA | 1 | Married | 4 | HH |
| Theresa Butler | 33 | 28 | White | CA | 2 | Married | 4 | HH |

* Class is defined as the combination of two characteristics: H(igh) education or L(ow) education (determined by whether or not the respondent earned a college degree), and H(igh) income or L(ow) income (determined by whether the respondent is financially eligible for WIC—having a household income above or below 185 percent of the federal poverty line).

## TABLE A.2. Mixed-Class Mothers

| Pseudonym | Age | Age at 1st Child | Race | State | Number of Children | Marital Status | 2011 Income Quintile | Class * |
|---|---|---|---|---|---|---|---|---|
| Annie Castro | 29 | 26 | White | FL | 2 | Married | 2 | HL |
| Cass Blackwell | 33 | 33 | White | FL | 1 | Married | 3 | LH |
| Christine Webber | 37 | 32 | White | FL | 3 | Married | 2 | HL |
| Dani Hahn | 24 | 23 | White | FL | 1 | Unmarried | 2 | LH |
| Dharma Wasserman | 48 | 41 | White | CA | 1 | Married | 5 | LH |
| Frankie Ford | 26 | 17 | White | FL | 3 | Married | 5 | LH |
| Gita Potter | 27 | 25 | Asian | CA | 1 | Married | 4 | HL |
| Ji-Eun Park | 35 | 29 | Asian | FL | 3 | Married | 2 | HL |
| Juana Reyes | 29 | 27 | Latina | CA | 1 | Married | 4 | HL |
| Kirsten Cooper | 38 | 34 | White | CA | 2 | Unmarried, cohabiting | 4 | LH |
| Lee Mendoza | 30 | 29 | White | CA | 1 | Married | 5 | HL |
| Louise Peralta | 36 | 34 | White | FL | 2 | Married | 3 | LH |
| Nicki Lindsay | 30 | 24 | White | FL | 2 | Married | 3 | HL |
| Noura Berry | 23 | 21 | White | FL | 1 | Unmarried | 2 | HL |

* Class is defined as the combination of two characteristics: H(igh) education or L(ow) education (determined by whether or not the respondent earned a college degree), and H(igh) income or L(ow) income (determined by whether the respondent is financially eligible for WIC—having a household income above or below 185 percent of the federal poverty line).

## Table A.3. Low-Education, Low-Income Mothers

| Pseudonym | Age | Age at 1st child | Race | State | Number of Children | Marital Status | 2011 Income Quintile | Class * |
|---|---|---|---|---|---|---|---|---|
| Becky Baker | 26 | 24 | White | CA | 2 | Married | 1 | LL |
| Chevonne Lewis | 23 | 21 | Black | FL | 2 | Unmarried, cohabiting | 2 | LL |
| Dawn Slade | 33 | 19 | White | FL | 8 | Married | 2 | LL |
| Gaby Romero | 29 | 29 | Latina | CA | 1 | Married | 2 | LL |
| Grace Kellogg | 20 | 20 | White | FL | 1 | Unmarried, cohabiting | 2 | LL |
| India Brown | 20 | 19 | Black | CA | 1 | Unmarried | 1 | LL |
| Janie Reed | 21 | 21 | Black | FL | 0 | Unmarried | 1 | LL |
| Jazmine Easton | 34 | 22 | Black | CA | 5 | Unmarried | 1 | LL |
| Jolene Ainsworth | 29 | 21 | White | FL | 3 | Married | 2 | LL |
| Kathryn Schmidt | 24 | 24 | White | FL | 1 | Unmarried | 2 | LL |
| Kiara Jefferson | 20 | 17 | Black | FL | 1 | Unmarried | 1 | LL |
| LaDonna Douglas | 18 | 18 | Black | FL | 1 | Unmarried, cohabiting | 1 | LL |
| Luz Flores | 28 | 17 | Latina | CA | 8 | Divorced | 1 | LL |
| Lynne O'Brien | 27 | 18 | White | FL | 3 | Married | 1 | LL |
| May Campbell | 40 | 20 | Black | FL | 3 | Married | 1 | LL |
| Mercedes Diaz | 19 | 18 | Latina | CA | 1 | Unmarried | 2 | LL |
| Nicole Johnson | 22 | 16 | Black | CA | 1 | Unmarried, cohabiting | 1 | LL |
| Patrice Martin | 36 | 19 | Black | FL | 4 | Unmarried | 1 | LL |
| Roberta Oakley | 25 | 23 | White | FL | 4 | Unmarried, cohabiting | 1 | LL |
| Rosa Acosta | 19 | 19 | Latina | CA | 1 | Unmarried | 1 | LL |
| Sarah Evans | 21 | 20 | White | FL | 1 | Unmarried | 1 | LL |
| Shawna Blanchard | 20 | 21 (anticipated) | Black | FL | 0 | Unmarried, cohabiting | 1 | LL |
| Shontel Sykes | 20 | 16 | Black | CA | 2 | Unmarried, cohabiting | 1 | LL |
| Tina Smith | 41 | 40 | Black | CA | 1 | Married | 1 | LL |
| Trisha Kent | 25 | 20 | White | FL | 2 | Married | 2 | LL |
| Vanessa Garfield | 25 | 21 | White | FL | 2 | Married | 2 | LL |

* Class is defined as the combination of two characteristics: H(igh) education or L(ow) education (determined by whether or not the respondent earned a college degree), and H(igh) income or L(ow) income (determined by whether the respondent is financially eligible for WIC—having a household income above or below 185 percent of the federal poverty line).

# NOTES

## INTRODUCTION

1 Throughout the book, I use the term "body care" to describe the work people do on their own or others' bodies. I use "body care" in place of "health care" because not all of these practices benefit health: some body care is health neutral (having more to do with, say, appearance than with well-being), and some body-care choices may even be harmful to health.

2 AAP 2012.

3 Oliveira et al. 2002.

4 Ehrenreich and English 2005; Fausto-Sterling 1992.

5 Buffington 2005; St. Louis 2003; Washington 2008; Waytz et al. 2012.

6 Bourdieu 1984, 190.

7 Fausto-Sterling 2005, 1495.

8 Bourdieu 1984, 175.

9 Bourdieu 1984, 192–93.

10 Bourdieu 1986, 5.

11 Parsons 1951.

12 Crawford 1980, 365.

13 Lupton 1995; Pelters and Wijma 2016.

14 Brown 2005, 42.

15 Crawford 1980.

16 Metzl 2010, 1–2.

17 I use the gendered term "maternal embodiment" with some ambivalence. While all of my participants are women, not everyone who experiences pregnancy and lactation is. In cases where transgender and nonbinary people share these experiences of heightened body consciousness and external surveillance, calling those experiences "maternal" would be inaccurate. At the same time, many of the social interactions participants describe are closely tied to their presentation as women: while feminine-presenting people with a protruding belly are likely to be "read" as pregnant (and thus subject to the mixture of protective and intrusive interactions that can entail), masculine-presenting pregnant people are more likely to be "read" as fat, exempting them from some pregnancy-related surveillance (see, for example, Hoffkling et al. 2017; Landau 2012).

18 McMillan Cottom 2019.

19 USDA 2011; Jones-Ellard 2010.

20  Centers for Disease Control (CDC) 2021; CDC 2010.

21  In 2010, this cutoff was equivalent to an annual income of $40,793 for a family of four.

22  While I occasionally reference my participant observation and interviews with WIC staff members throughout the book, they mostly serve to provide context for the interviews with mothers that form the core of this book's data. For articles that draw more directly on my conversations with WIC staff, see Mason 2016a and Mason 2016b.

23  Tax Policy Center 2020.

24  For a discussion of why health researchers often examine class as a function of both education and income, see, for example, Pamela Herd et al. 2007 and Gabriela J. Oates et al. 2017. Herd and colleagues find that "education is more predictive than income of the *onset* of both functional limitations and chronic conditions, while income is more strongly associated than education with the *progression* of both" (223). They also note that educational differences are more associated with class differences in health behaviors, whereas income differences matter insofar as they mediate individuals' access to resources.

25  Lareau 2003.

26  DiMaggio and Mohr 1985.

27  Jack 2019.

28  Craig 2021.

29  Bridges 2020; Mude et al. 2021; Williams 2012.

30  Braveman et al. 20121; Marmot and Wilkinson 2005.

## CHAPTER 1. MATERNAL EMBODIMENT

1  Throughout the book, I will use the following shorthand to denote mothers' class positions: HH=high-education, high-income; LL=low-education, low-income. Mixed-class mothers were either HL (high-education, low-income) or LH (low-education, high-income).

2  Foucault 1995.

3  For further discussion of the privacy tradeoffs that people receiving public assistance often have to make, see Mason 2016a; McCormack 2005; Randles and Woodward 2018.

4  Shilling 1993, 6–7.

5  Conrad, 1992; Zola 1972.

6  Mayo Clinic 2018.

7  Khazan 2014.

8  Lareau 2003, 129.

9  Aquilino and Supple 1991; Arnett 2000; Padilla-Walker et al. 2012.

10  Livingston 2015: "For most highly educated women, motherhood doesn't start until the 30s."

11  Kelly 2013; Malamud and Wozniak 2010.

12  Jones and Buttenheim 2014; Pearlstein 2019.

13 Wu 2021; Zipprich et al. 2015.

14 Reich 2016.

15 While it is possible that Nicole actually did have several biological/legally related cousins who all became pregnant around the same time, it is more likely that she was referring to "play cousins"—close family friends and neighbors who become fictive kin, particularly within some Black communities. See The Root Staff 2014 for more on this practice.

16 For example, see Hays 1996.

17 Pew Research Center 2015.

## CHAPTER 2. THE GENDER OF WELLNESS

1 DeVault 1994, 116.

2 Hochschild and Machung 2012.

3 Thébaud and colleagues tested the popular myth of male "dirt blindness," which posits that men are not avoiding housework; they just have an inability to see mess. The study found that men and women did not substantially differ in their evaluations when shown an image of a clean or messy room. This supports Hochschild and Machung's contention that "I don't see dirt" is a strategy—employed more often by men—to avoid responsibility for housework rather than a statement of fact.

4 American Academy of Allergy, Asthma & Immunology 2020.

5 Penha-Lopes 2006; Berridge and Romich 2011.

6 Sayer and Fine 2011, 264.

7 Stalsberg and Pedersen 2018; Monsivais et al. 2014; Daniel 2016.

8 Bowen et al. 2019.

9 Cowan 1985; Hays 1996; Strasser 2000.

10 Bordo 2004, 160.

11 The linkages among bodies, gender, control, sexuality, and eating disorders have been extensively documented. Susan Bordo (2004) cites the cases of several anorexic patients who tied slenderness to asexuality: "staying reed-thin is seen as a way of avoiding sexuality"; and the "dread of gaining weight [stems from] 'not wanting to be a temptation to men'" (148). Other women may turn to binge eating in the wake of an assault in an attempt to "deflect sexual attention" and as a source of pleasure "to anesthetize a multitude of 'negative' feelings" (Root 1991, 98).

12 Womenshealth.gov resources on sexual assault and rape.

13 Young 1990.

14 Official rules for a variety of sports, both past and present, have treated women's bodies as more fragile and less capable than men's. The long-standing ban on women in the Boston Marathon, which only officially ended in 1972, is one example; more recently, the exclusion of women's ski jumping events from the Winter Olympic Games until 2014, due in part to pseudoscientific concerns about risks to women's reproductive organs, is another. See Mooallem 2018.

15 Martin 1998.

16  Ferguson 2020.
17  Young 1990, 148.
18  Metzl 2010, 1–2.
19  Peralta 2007, 741.
20  Contois 2020; Courtenay 2000; Moore 2010; Petrzela 2017.
21  Saltonstall 1993; West and Zimmerman 1987; Williams 2000.
22  Williams 2000, 392.
23  West and Zimmerman 1987, 136.
24  Bordo 2004, 143.
25  Beauvoir 2012.
26  DeVault 1994, 113.
27  Murkoff and Mazel 2005, 90.
28  MacKendrick 2018.
29  Lupton 1999, 60.
30  Waggoner 2017, 27. See also Waggoner 2015.
31  Roberts 1997; Hankin et al. 1998.
32  MacKendrick 2018, 18.
33  Paul 2010.
34  Paul 2010.
35  This section draws on ethnographic observations and staff interviews I conducted at offices of the WIC program in California and Florida. For a fuller discussion of the processes of state-sponsored responsibilization, empowerment, and control I observed in these settings, see Mason 2016a and 2016b.
36  Reich 2012.

## CHAPTER 3. THE COSTS OF AVOIDING RISK

1  Apple 1995.
2  MacKendrick 2018.
3  Zelizer 1994.
4  Colen and Ramey 2014; LaFrance 2015; Senapathy 2016.
5  Blum 1999.
6  Hausman 2003, 6.
7  National Institutes of Health 2018.
8  Bourdieu 1984, 195.
9  Gleason et al. 2020.
10  See Laura Harrison's article "What's Best for Baby?" for an in-depth discussion of the public-awareness campaigns against bed sharing.
11  Oster 2013, xxii.
12  Boston Women's Health Book Collective 2011; Ehrenreich and English 2005.
13  Jetelina 2022. Jetelina, a mother of two young children, discusses how she began the project in a 2022 *Medscape* podcast with Dr. Eric Topol (Topol et al. 2022).
14  North 2021.
15  Queen 2016.

16 Freeborn 2018.

17 Apple 1995, 161.

18 Boehmová 2018; Momigliano 2019.

19 MacKendrick 2018.

20 "Attachment parenting," popularized by the series of books by Dr. Sears and his colleagues, advocates keeping babies and toddlers physically close to their caregivers via "baby-wearing" (using a wrap or infant carrier), breastfeeding, and cosleeping. "Elimination communication" is an approach some parents use to avoid diapering infants and toddlers, which depends on caregivers becoming attuned to a child's physical signs that indicate the need to urinate or defecate, then bringing the child to a toilet or bowl where they can take care of their elimination needs. Both of these approaches require a parent—usually a mother—to be physically close to the child virtually all of the time. Needless to say, these approaches are incompatible with most paid work in the contemporary United States.

21 Blum 1993, 300.

22 Williams et al. 2015.

23 Newman 2012; Nicholls 2016.

24 Ashley Fetters (2020) traces the rise of the "wine mom" meme to the mid-2010s, when it "became commonplace for moms to joke online about drinking wine to cope with the stresses of motherhood." On one hand, the cultural figure of the "wine mom" becomes a way for mothers to acknowledge that parenting is hard work, and to appear slightly less angelic than motherhood ideals typically allow for. On the other hand, as Ashley Abramson (2018) points out, this trope also normalizes heavy alcohol use among women while glossing over a real need for postpartum care and societal support for primary caregivers.

25 Lightdale and Gremse 2013.

26 Edwards et al. 2021; Roberts 2002.

27 Lupton 1993, 427.

28 Waggoner 2017.

29 Ladd-Taylor and Umansky 1998, 3.

30 Daniels 1997, 582.

### CHAPTER 4. THE STORIES MOTHERS TELL

1 "Crunchy granola" is a slang term, originating in the 1970s United States, to describe someone as a "hippie." The term typically connotes someone who is politically liberal, environmentally conscious, and devoted to making and consuming health foods.

2 Attachment parenting, recall, is a time-intensive approach that claims to foster secure emotional attachment in children by encouraging close physical contact between parents and children; practitioners often describe this method as the most "natural" or "intuitive" way to parent, though there are also countless books, websites, and consumer goods devoted to teaching people how to practice attachment parenting. See, for example, askdrsears.com (Sears 2020).

3 In her discussion of "stone age mothering," Bernice Hausman (2003) deconstructs the rhetorics of evolutionary, primal, or "caveman"-style health and parenting advice. As she explains, focusing on the case of breastfeeding, "Evolution is brought into breastfeeding advocacy as a way to argue for and rationalize particular breast-feeding behaviors in the context of *idealized familial arrangements* (the middle-class, nuclear family in which the wife-mother stays at home and the husband-father earns a living in the paid labor force) and *idealized stereotypes of mothering* (mother as sacrificial figure who lovingly negates her personal needs or desires in service to her children)" (126). Similarly, "primal" eating, "attachment parenting," and the like are time- and body-intensive health regimens that encourage people—usually mothers—to eschew modern conveniences like prepackaged food or paid childcare, ostensibly in the interest of their own or their child's well-being.

4 Giddens 1991, 5.

5 Giddens 1991, 52.

6 Bailey 1999.

7 See Waggoner 2012.

8 At the time of this writing, the American College of Obstetricians and Gynecologists recommended that pregnant people aim for 150 minutes of moderate aerobic activity per week, offering examples such as gardening or brisk walking.

9 Bridges 2011, 45–46.

10 Smith 1974, 10. See also Hughes (1945) and Levy et al. (2002) for further discussion of motherhood as a "master status."

11 Muñoz 2013, 11.

12 Hare Krishna (or, ISKCON—the International Society for Krishna Consciousness) does not take an official stance on vaccines and other forms of modern medicine. Devotees are urged to be thoughtful about what they put into their bodies—for example, committed members are expected to abstain from eating meat, fish, and eggs—and while many seek out vaccines and other affordances of Western/allopathic medicine, other practitioners are skeptical of modern medicine, preferring complementary and alternative medicine. Thus, while Noura viewed her vaccine refusal as an expression of her religious faith, that choice was not dictated by the society's governing body: it was, rather, her own interpretation of the faith's precepts, shaped by her own values and priorities.

13 Dow 2016, 181.

14 Tinsley 2018.

15 Giddens 1991.

16 Bourdieu 1984.

17 See Caitlin Daniel (2016) for further evidence about the ways economic constraint and early childhood dietary patterns shape tastes later in life

## CHAPTER 5. RIGID AND FLEXIBLE AGENCY

1 Bordo 2004, 247.

2 Benson 1990, 49.

3 Benson 1990, 50.

4 Mahmood 2001, 207.

5 See, for example, Fausto-Sterling 1992; Shildrick 2015; and Fischer 1992.

6 Shildrick 2015, 26.

7 Bordo 2004, 9.

8 Strings 2019, 6–7.

9 Strings 2019, 116.

10 Strings 2019, 100.

11 Bourdieu 1984, 192–93.

12 Young 1990, 160.

13 Benson 1990, 50.

14 While this bodily sensation of containing another being within oneself is common in pregnancy, especially once the fetus's kicks and movements become apparent, it does not follow that every pregnant person perceives that being as a *person*. Some also, variably, conceptualize their womb's current occupant as a parasite, alien, or other not-quite-human being (even when the pregnancy is desired).

15 Mahmood 2012, 5.

16 Mahmood 2012, 14–15.

17 Denbow 2005, 221.

18 Dow 2016, 185.

19 Randles 2021, 7.

20 Denbow 2005.

21 Wolf 2003, 86.

22 Nelson 1982, 349.

23 Lazarus 1994, 25.

24 Epstein 2008; Gaskin 2010.

25 Gifford et al. 2017.

26 Bridges 2011.

27 Holgash and Heberlein 2019.

28 Aizer et al. 2007; Gray 2001.

29 Johnson and Simon 2021.

30 Villarosa 2018.

31 Centers for Disease Control (CDC) 2016.

32 Lareau 2003.

33 Asbring 2001; Bury 1982.

34 Charmaz 1994; Williams 2000.

35 Levy et al. 2002.

36 Siebers 2016, 315–16.

## CHAPTER 6. CARE WORK AS STATUS WORK

1 Emily's emphasis on eating "real," home-cooked food is likewise a subtle marker of class privilege. As Sarah Bowen, Joslyn Brenton, and Sinikka Elliott argue in

*Pressure Cooker*, the supposed health and budgetary benefits of home cooking are overstated. Pollan's rules assume that families—usually mothers—will have adequate time, equipment, knowledge, storage, and more to prepare the sort of healthful meals he celebrates. See also Gordon and Hobbes 2022.

2  Laurison et al. 2020.

3  Lamont and Small 2008, 86.

4  Lareau 2003, 39.

5  Lareau 2003, 67.

6  Willis 2017.

7  Lamont 2012, 1.

8  See, for example, Jennifer Randles's discussion of poverty, diaper need, and dignity in "Willing to Do Anything for My Kids" (2021), as well as Dorothy Roberts's discussion of the disproportionate policing of low-income and Black children's health and hygiene in *Shattered Bonds* (2002).

9  Mani et al. 2013.

10  The links between low socioeconomic status and high rates of chronic illness—also known as the "social determinants of health"—are well established, but Gabriela Oates et al. (2017) offer a helpful overview of the range of conditions linked to socioeconomic status and racial disparities, as well as differentiating between the effects of income and education on health.

11  Lareau 2003.

12  Willis 2017.

13  Bourdieu 1984.

14  Bills 2003; Friedman and Laurison 2019.

15  Brady 2004.

16  Pascoe 2011.

17  Messerschmidt 2011.

18  Crandall 1991, 1995.

19  Cook 2017; Park 2019.

20  Mason 2012.

21  Biddle and Hamermesh 1998; Riniolo et al. 2006. For a nationally representative sample looking at the earnings disparities among people rated as more or less physically attractive, see Monk et al. 2021.

22  Barber 2021, 245.

23  Westwood 2018.

24  See also Frankel 2015.

25  Stempel 2005, 428.

## CONCLUSION

1  See, for example, Cutler and Lleras-Muney (2006) for evidence that education—and not merely the socioeconomic benefits it confers—improves health.

2  According to research by Caitlin Daniel, who argues that children might need ten or more exposures to a new food before they develop a taste for it, the fear of food

waste is a significant factor in low-income parents' decisions about how and what to feed their children.

3  Ehrenreich 2014.

4  For another example of public health campaigns that target individual behavior, rather than structural inequalities (and in doing so implicitly frame poor and racial/ethnic minority women as bad mothers), see Laura Harrison's (2018) discussion of Milwaukee's "Safe Sleep Campaign," which aimed to reduce infant mortality in low-income communities by discouraging bed sharing.

5  Daniel Kim and Adrianna Saada's article, "The Social Determinants of Infant Mortality and Birth Outcomes in Western Developed Nations" (2013), offers a longer, cross-national discussion of the social determinants of infant mortality and birth outcomes.

6  WIC, of course, did offer free food as well as referrals to other social-assistance programs that could help clients access healthcare, affordable housing, and subsidies for utility bills. But it is worth noting that the average monthly value of WIC's food vouchers in 2008 was $43.40/person. It spent $41.10 per person—almost an additional month's worth of food—for the year on education (FNS 2010). For reference, in 2012, the median household spent about $125/week on food—a little over $500/month (Mendes 2012).

   To be clear, this financial help mattered to many households (women told me how much they appreciated having the extra space in their household food budgets made possible by WIC vouchers), but WIC also could have done more: provide more food options, including covering organics and other specialized products, and more dollar value in what it covered. And many women noted that the benefits of WIC needed to be weighed against the time and energy it took to attend appointments, travel to and from the office, sit in the waiting room, and wait on hold to speak to someone if they needed to reschedule an appointment.

7  Bourdieu 1984.

8  Mani et al. 2013, 980.

9  Ruiz et al. 2015.

10  Mani et al. 2013.

11  For an example of an innovative program that uses doulas to advocate for disadvantaged laboring mothers in healthcare settings, see Marilyn C. Moses and Roberto Hugh Potter, "The Use of Doulas for Inmates in Labor" (2008).

12  Cowan 1985; Strasser 2000.

13  Hays 1996; Lareau 2003.

14  See Dow 2016; and Riché J. Daniel Barnes's concept of "strategic mothering" in *Raising the Race* (2015).

15  Suzanne Bianchi et al.'s "Housework" (2012), along with their earlier "Is Anyone Doing the Housework?" (2000), both demonstrate the persistent gender gap in household responsibility for household labor. This gap narrowed as a result of the women's movement but plateaued, and gender differences in the *type* of house-

hold labor married spouses were doing show that women are responsible for more routine, nonnegotiable tasks like feeding, while men perform more sporadic and discretionary chores like mowing the lawn. Liana C. Sayer and Leigh Fine's article, "Racial-Ethnic Differences in U.S. Married Women's and Men's Housework" (2011), and Erik Olin Wright et al.'s "Non-Effects of Class on the Gender Division of Labor in the Home" (1992), explore racial and class variations in the size of the gender gap in housework. While Wright and colleagues found little significant class variation, Sayer and Fine found that Hispanic and Asian women did more "core housework" than did Black and white women, but there was very little racial/ethnic variation in men's participation in core housework.

16 Garland-Thomson 2002, 5.

17 See, for example, Richard Wilkinson and Kate Pickett's *Spirit Level* (2011) and the documentary series *Unnatural Causes* for details on the multiple ways in which social inequality itself—not just poverty—harms overall societal health and well-being.

18 Tegan Cruwys et al. 2016.

# REFERENCES

Abramson, Ashley. 2018. "The Cheeky 'Wine Mom' Trope Isn't Just Dumb. It's Dangerous." *Washington Post*, September 21.

Adelman, Larry. 2008. *Unnatural Causes: Is Inequality Making Us Sick?* Produced by California Newsreel with Vital Pictures Inc. www.unnaturalcauses.org.

Aizer, Anna, Janet Currie, and Enrico Moretti. 2007. "Does Managed Care Hurt Health? Evidence from Medicaid Mothers." *Review of Economics and Statistics* 89(3):385–99. doi: 10.1162/rest.89.3.385.

American Academy of Allergy, Asthma, and Immunology. 2020. "Prevention of Allergies and Asthma in Children." Retrieved March 4, 2022. www.aaaai.org.

American Academy of Pediatrics (AAP). 2012. "Breastfeeding and the Use of Human Milk." *Pediatrics* 129(3):e827–41. doi: 10.1542/peds.2011–3552.

Apple, Rima D. 1995. "Constructing Mothers: Scientific Motherhood in the Nineteenth and Twentieth Centuries." *Social History of Medicine* 8(2):161–78. doi: 10.1093/shm/8.2.161.

Aquilino, William S., and Khalil R. Supple. 1991. "Parent-Child Relations and Parents' Satisfaction with Living Arrangements When Adult Children Live at Home." *Journal of Marriage and Family* 53(1):13–27. doi: 10.2307/353130.

Arnett, Jeffrey Jensen. 2000. "Emerging Adulthood: A Theory of Development from the Late Teens through the Twenties." *American Psychologist* 55(5):469–80. doi: 10.1037/0003–066X.55.5.469.

Asbring, Pia. 2001. "Chronic Illness—a Disruption in Life: Identity-Transformation among Women with Chronic Fatigue Syndrome and Fibromyalgia." *Journal of Advanced Nursing* 34(3):312–19. doi: 10.1046/j.1365–2648.2001.01767.x.

Bailey, Lucy. 1999. "Refracted Selves? A Study of Changes in Self-Identity in the Transition to Motherhood." *Sociology* 33(2):335–52.

Barber, Kristen. 2021. "Good-Looking Men Require Hard-Working Women: The Labor of Consumption in the Grooming Industry." In *The Oxford Handbook of the Sociology of Body and Embodiment*, edited by N. Boero and K. Mason. Oxford University Press.

Barnes, Riché J. Daniel. 2015. *Raising the Race: Black Career Women Redefine Marriage, Motherhood, and Community*. Rutgers University Press.

Beauvoir, Simone de. 2012. *The Second Sex*. Knopf Doubleday.

Benson, Paul. 1990. "Feminist Second Thoughts about Free Agency." *Hypatia* 5(3):47–64. doi: 10.1111/j.1527–2001.1990.tb00605.x.

Berridge, Clara W., and Jennifer L. Romich. 2011. "'Raising Him . . . to Pull His Own Weight': Boys' Household Work in Single-Mother Households." *Journal of Family Issues* 32(2):157–80. doi: 10.1177/0192513X10380832.

Bianchi, Suzanne M., Melissa A. Milkie, Liana C. Sayer, and John P. Robinson. 2000. "Is Anyone Doing the Housework? Trends in the Gender Division of Household Labor." *Social Forces* 79(1):191–228. doi: 10.2307/2675569.

Bianchi, Suzanne M., Liana C. Sayer, Melissa A. Milkie, and John P. Robinson. 2012. "Housework: Who Did, Does, or Will Do It, and How Much Does It Matter?" *Social Forces* 91(1):55–63. doi: 10.1093/sf/sos120.

Biddle, Jeff E., and Daniel S. Hamermesh. 1998. "Beauty, Productivity, and Discrimination: Lawyers' Looks and Lucre." *Journal of Labor Economics* 16(1):172–201. doi: 10.1086/209886.

Bills, David B. 2003. "Credentials, Signals, and Screens: Explaining the Relationship between Schooling and Job Assignment." *Review of Educational Research* 73(4):441–69. doi: 10.3102/00346543073004441.

Blum, Linda M. 1993. "Mothers, Babies, and Breastfeeding in Late Capitalist America: The Shifting Contexts of Feminist Theory." *Feminist Studies* 19(2):291.

———. 1999. *At the Breast: Ideologies of Breastfeeding and Motherhood in the Contemporary United States.* Beacon Press.

Boehmová, Zuzana. 2018. "The Cost and Value of Breast Milk." *Slate Magazine*, February 13.

Bordo, Susan. 2004. *Unbearable Weight: Feminism, Western Culture, and the Body.* University of California Press.

Boston Women's Health Book Collective and Judy Norsigian. 2011. *Our Bodies, Ourselves.* Touchstone.

Bourdieu, Pierre. 1984. *Distinction: A Social Critique of the Judgement of Taste.* Harvard University Press.

———. 1986. "The Forms of Capital." Pp. 241–58 in *Handbook of Theory and Research for the Sociology of Education*, edited by J. Richardson. Greenwood.

Bowen, Sarah, Joslyn Brenton, and Sinikka Elliott. 2019. *Pressure Cooker: Why Home Cooking Won't Solve Our Problems and What We Can Do about It.* Oxford University Press.

Brady, Patrick. 2004. "Jocks, Teckers, and Nerds: The Role of the Adolescent Peer Group in the Formation and Maintenance of Secondary School Institutional Culture." *Discourse: Studies in the Cultural Politics of Education* 25(3):351–64. doi: 10.1080/0159630042000247926.

Braveman, Paula, Susan Egerter, and David R. Williams. 2011. "The Social Determinants of Health: Coming of Age." *Annual Review of Public Health* 32(1):381–98. doi: 10.1146/annurev-publhealth-031210-101218.

Bridges, Khiara. 2011. *Reproducing Race: An Ethnography of Pregnancy as a Site of Racialization.* University of California Press.

———. 2020. "Racial Disparities in Maternal Mortality." *New York University Law Review* 95:1229.

Brown, Wendy. 2005. *Edgework: Critical Essays on Knowledge and Politics*. Princeton University Press.

Buffington, Daniel. 2005. "Contesting Race on Sundays: Making Meaning out of the Rise in the Number of Black Quarterbacks." *Sociology of Sport Journal* 22(1):19–37.

Bury, Michael. 1982. "Chronic Illness as Biographical Disruption." *Sociology of Health & Illness* 4(2):167–82. doi: 10.1111/1467–9566.ep11339939.

CDC. 2010. "Breastfeeding Report Card: United States, 2010," p. 4. CDC. www.cdc.gov. Retrieved October 9, 2022.

———. 2016. "Racial and Ethnic Disparities Continue in Pregnancy-Related Deaths: Black, American Indian/Alaska Native Women Most Affected." CDC. Retrieved August 27, 2021. www.cdc.gov.

———. 2021. "Maternity Practices in Infant Nutrition and Care (MPINC) Survey." CDC. Retrieved August 17, 2021. www.cdc.gov.

Charmaz, Kathy. 1994. "Identity Dilemmas of Chronically Ill Men." *Sociological Quarterly* 35(2):269–88. doi: 10.1111/j.1533–8525.1994.tb00410.x.

Colen, Cynthia G., and David M. Ramey. 2014. "Is Breast Truly Best? Estimating the Effects of Breastfeeding on Long-Term Child Health and Wellbeing in the United States Using Sibling Comparisons." *Social Science & Medicine* 109:55–65. doi: 10.1016/j.socscimed.2014.01.027.

Conrad, Peter. 1992. "Medicalization and Social Control." *Annual Review of Sociology* 18:209–32.

Contois, Emily J. H. 2020. *Diners, Dudes, and Diets: How Gender and Power Collide in Food Media and Culture*. University of North Carolina Press.

Cook, Bob. 2017. "Using Sports to Get Out of Poverty Doesn't Work When You Have to Be Rich to Play." *Forbes*, March 25. www.forbes.com.

Courtenay, Will H. 2000. "Constructions of Masculinity and Their Influence on Men's Well-Being: A Theory of Gender and Health." *Social Science & Medicine* 50(10):1385–1401. doi: 10.1016/S0277–9536(99)00390–1.

Cowan, Ruth Schwartz. 1985. *More Work for Mother: The Ironies of Household Technology from the Open Hearth to the Microwave*. Basic Books.

Craig, Maxine Leeds. 2021. "Methodologies for Categories in Motion." In *The Oxford Handbook of the Sociology of Body and Embodiment*, edited by N. Boero and K. Mason. Oxford University Press.

Crandall, Christian S. 1991. "Do Heavy-Weight Students Have More Difficulty Paying for College?" *Personality and Social Psychology Bulletin* 17(6):606–11.

———. 1995. "Do Parents Discriminate against Their Heavyweight Daughters?" *Personality and Social Psychology Bulletin* 21(7):724–35. doi: 10.1177/0146167295217007.

Crawford, Robert. 1980. "Healthism and the Medicalization of Everyday Life." *International Journal of Health Services* 10(3):365–88.

Cruwys, Tegan, Carly T. Leverington, and Anne M. Sheldon. 2016. "An Experimental Investigation of the Consequences and Social Functions of Fat Talk in Friendship Groups." *International Journal of Eating Disorders* 49(1):84–91. doi: 10.1002/eat.22446.

Cutler, David M., and Adriana Lleras-Muney. 2006. *Education and Health: Evaluating Theories and Evidence.* Working Paper 12352. National Bureau of Economic Research. doi: 10.3386/w12352.

Daniel, Caitlin. 2016. "Economic Constraints on Taste Formation and the True Cost of Healthy Eating." *Social Science & Medicine* 148:34–41. doi: 10.1016/j.socscimed.2015.11.025.

Daniels, Cynthia R. 1997. "Between Fathers and Fetuses: The Social Construction of Male Reproduction and the Politics of Fetal Harm." *Signs* 22(3):579–616.

Denbow, Jennifer. 2005. "Abortion: When Choice and Autonomy Conflict; Recent Developments." *Berkeley Journal of Gender, Law & Justice* 20(1):216–28.

DeVault, Marjorie L. 1994. *Feeding the Family: The Social Organization of Caring as Gendered Work.* University of Chicago Press.

DiMaggio, Paul, and John Mohr. 1985. "Cultural Capital, Educational Attainment, and Marital Selection." *American Journal of Sociology* 90(6):1231–61.

Dow, Dawn Marie. 2016. "Integrated Motherhood: Beyond Hegemonic Ideologies of Motherhood." *Journal of Marriage and Family* 78(1):180–96. doi: 10.1111/jomf.12264.

Edwards, Frank, Sara Wakefield, Kieran Healy, and Christopher Wildeman. 2021. "Contact with Child Protective Services Is Pervasive but Unequally Distributed by Race and Ethnicity in Large US Counties." *Proceedings of the National Academy of Sciences* 118(30):e2106272118. doi: 10.1073/pnas.2106272118.

Ehrenreich, Barbara. 2014. "It Is Expensive to Be Poor." *Atlantic*, January 13. www.theatlantic.com.

Ehrenreich, Barbara, and Deirdre English. 2005. *Witches, Midwives, and Nurses: A History of Women Healers.* Black Powder Press.

Epstein, Abby, dir. 2008. *The Business of Being Born.* Netflix.

Fausto-Sterling, Anne. 1992. *Myths of Gender: Biological Theories about Women and Men.* 2nd ed. Basic Books.

———. 2005. "The Bare Bones of Sex: Part 1—Sex and Gender." *Signs: Journal of Women in Culture and Society* 30(2):1491–1527. doi: 10.1086/424932.

———. 2008. *Myths of Gender: Biological Theories about Women and Men.* Rev. ed. Basic Books.

Ferguson, Ann Arnett. 2020. *Bad Boys: Public Schools in the Making of Black Masculinity.* University of Michigan Press.

Fetters, Ashley. 2020. "The Many Faces of the 'Wine Mom.'" *Atlantic*, May 23. www.theatlantic.com.

Fischer, Lucy. 1992. "Birth Traumas: Parturition and Horror in 'Rosemary's Baby.'" *Cinema Journal* 31(3):3–18. doi: 10.2307/1225505.

Food and Nutrition Service Office of Research and Analysis (FNS). 2010. *Nutrition Education and Promotion: The Role of FNS in Helping Low-Income Families Make Healthier Eating and Lifestyle Choices. A Report to Congress.* www.fns.usda.gov.

Foucault, Michel. 1995. *Discipline and Punish: The Birth of the Prison.* Knopf Doubleday.

Frakt, Austin. 2019. "Does Your Education Level Affect Your Health?" *New York Times*, June 3.

Frankel, Ryan. 2015. "Why You Should Hire Athletes." *Forbes*, September 30. www. forbes.com.

Freeborn, T. 2018. "Confirmation Bias." Customer review of *Expecting Better: Why the Conventional Pregnancy Wisdom Is Wrong—and What You Really Need to Know*, by Emily Oster. Amazon. Retrieved August 25, 2021. www.amazon.com.

Friedman, Sam, and Daniel Laurison. 2019. *The Class Ceiling: Why It Pays to Be Privileged*. Policy Press.

Garland-Thomson, Rosemarie. 2002. "Integrating Disability, Transforming Feminist Theory." *NWSA Journal* 14(3):1–32.

Gaskin, Ina May. 2010. *Spiritual Midwifery*. Book Publishing Company.

Giddens, Anthony. 1991. *Modernity and Self-Identity: Self and Society in the Late Modern Age*. Stanford University Press.

Gifford, Kathy, Jenna Walls, Usha Ranji, and Ivette Gomez. 2017. "Medicaid Coverage of Pregnancy and Perinatal Benefits: Results from a State Survey." Kaiser Family Foundation. Retrieved August 27, 2021. www.kff.org.

Gleason, Jessica, Fasil Tekola-Ayele, Rajeshwari Sundaram, Stefanie N. Hinkle, Yassaman Vafai, Germaine M. Buck Louis, Nicole Gerlanc, Melissa Amyx, Alaina M. Bever, Melissa M. Smarr, Morgan Robinson, Kurunthachalam Kannan, and Katherine L. Grantz. 2021. "Association between Maternal Caffeine Consumption and Metabolism and Neonatal Anthropometry: A Secondary Analysis of the NICHD Fetal Growth Studies–Singletons." *JAMA Network Open* 4(3):e213238. doi: 10.1001/jamanetworkopen.2021.3238.

Gordon, Aubrey, and Michael Hobbes. 2022. "Maintenance Phase: Michael Pollan's *The Omnivore's Dilemma* on Apple Podcasts." Apple Podcasts, April 5. https://podcasts. apple.com.

Gray, Bradley. 2001. "Do Medicaid Physician Fees for Prenatal Services Affect Birth Outcomes?" *Journal of Health Economics* 20(4):571–90. doi: 10.1016/S0167-6296(01)00085-6.

Hankin, Janet R., James J. Sloan, and Robert J. Sokol. 1998. "The Modest Impact of the Alcohol Beverage Warning Label on Drinking during Pregnancy among a Sample of African-American Women." *Journal of Public Policy & Marketing* 17(1):61–69.

Harrison, Laura. 2018. "What's Best for Baby? Co-sleeping and the Politics of Inequality." *Frontiers: A Journal of Women Studies* 39(3):63–95. doi: 10.5250/fronjwomestud.39.3.0063.

Hausman, Bernice L. 2003. *Mother's Milk: Breastfeeding Controversies in American Culture*. Psychology Press.

Hays, Sharon. 1996. *The Cultural Contradictions of Motherhood*. Yale University Press.

Herd, Pamela, Brian Goesling, and James S. House. 2007. "Socioeconomic Position and Health: The Differential Effects of Education versus Income on the Onset versus Progression of Health Problems." *Journal of Health and Social Behavior* 48(3):223–38. doi: 10.1177/002214650704800302.

Hochschild, Arlie, and Anne Machung. 2012. *The Second Shift: Working Families and the Revolution at Home*. Penguin.

Hoffkling, Alexis, Juno Obedin-Maliver, and Jae Sevelius. 2017. "From Erasure to Opportunity: A Qualitative Study of the Experiences of Transgender Men around Pregnancy and Recommendations for Providers." *BMC Pregnancy Childbirth* 17(332).

Holgash, Kayla, and Martha Heberlein. 2019. *Physician Acceptance of New Medicaid Patients*. Medicaid and CHIP Payment and Access Commission.

Hughes, Everett Cherrington. 1945. "Dilemmas and Contradictions of Status." *American Journal of Sociology* 50(5):353–59. doi: 10.1086/219652.

Jack, Anthony Abraham. 2019. *The Privileged Poor: How Elite Colleges Are Failing Disadvantaged Students*. Harvard University Press.

Jetelina, Katelyn. 2022. "Long COVID Mini-Series: Kids." *Your Local Epidemiologist*, March 9. https://yourlocalepidemiologist.substack.com.

Johnson, Katherine M., and Richard M. Simon. 2021. "Privilege in the Delivery Room? Race, Class, and the Realization of Natural Birth Preferences, 2002–2013." *Social Problems* 68(3):552–73. doi: 10.1093/socpro/spaa013.

Jones, Malia, and Alison Buttenheim. 2014. "Potential Effects of California's New Vaccine Exemption Law on the Prevalence and Clustering of Exemptions." *American Journal of Public Health* 104(9):e3–6. doi: 10.2105/AJPH.2014.302065.

Jones-Ellard, Sam. 2010. "USDA Highlights Nearly 900 Operating Winter Farmers Markets: Many Markets Located in Cold-Weather States." USDA Agricultural Marketing Service. ams.usda.gov.

Kelly, Brian. 2013. "The Process of Socio-Economic Constraint on Geographical Mobility: England 1991 to 2008." The Cathie Marsh Centre for Census and Survey Research. www.cmi.manchester.ac.uk.

Khazan, Olga. 2014. "Why Are There So Few Doctors in Rural America?" *Atlantic*, August 28.

Kim, Daniel, and Adrianna Saada. 2013. "The Social Determinants of Infant Mortality and Birth Outcomes in Western Developed Nations: A Cross-Country Systematic Review." *International Journal of Environmental Research and Public Health* 10(6):2296–2335. doi: 10.3390/ijerph10062296.

Ladd-Taylor, Molly, and Lauri Umansky, eds. 1998. *Bad Mothers: The Politics of Blame in Twentieth-Century America*. NYU Press.

LaFrance, Adrienne. 2015. "About That Breastfeeding Study." *Atlantic*, March 20. www.theatlantic.com.

Lamont, Michèle. 2012. *Money, Morals, and Manners: The Culture of the French and the American Upper-Middle Class*. University of Chicago Press.

Lamont, Michèle, and Mario Luis Small. 2008. "How Culture Matters: Enriching Our Understandings of Poverty." Pp. 76–102 in *The Colors of Poverty: Why Racial and Ethnic Disparities Persist*, edited by D. Harris and A. Lin. Russell Sage Foundation.

Landau, Jamie. 2012. "Reproducing and Transgressing Masculinity: A Rhetorical Analysis of Women Interacting with Digital Photographs of Thomas Beatie." *Women's Studies in Communication* 35(2):178–203.

Lareau, Annette. 2003. *Unequal Childhoods: Class, Race, and Family Life*. University of California Press.

Laurison, Daniel, Dawn Dow, and Carolyn Chernoff. 2020. "Class Mobility and Reproduction for Black and White Adults in the United States: A Visualization." *Socius*, January. doi: 10.1177/2378023120960959.

Lazarus, Ellen S. 1994. "What Do Women Want? Issues of Choice, Control, and Class in Pregnancy and Childbirth." *Medical Anthropology Quarterly* 8(1):25–46.

Levy, Becca, Martin Slade, and Stanislav Kasl. 2002. "Longevity Increased by Positive Self-Perceptions of Aging." *Journal of Personality and Social Psychology* 83:261–70. doi: 10.1037/0022-3514.83.2.261.

Levy, René, Eric Widmer, and Jean Kellerhals. 2002. "Modern Family or Modernized Family Traditionalism? Master Status and the Gender Order in Switzerland." *Electronic Journal of Sociology* 6(4).

Lightdale, Jenifer, and David Gremse. 2013. "Gastroesophageal Reflux: Management Guidance for the Pediatrician." *Pediatrics* 131(5):e1684–95. doi: 10.1542/peds.2013-0421.

Livingston, Gretchen. 2015. *For Most Highly Educated Women, Motherhood Doesn't Start until the 30s*. Pew Research Center.

Lupton, Deborah. 1993. "Risk as Moral Danger: The Social and Political Functions of Risk Discourse in Public Health." *International Journal of Health Services* 23(3):425–35. doi: 10.2190/16AY-E2GC-DFLD-51X2.

———. 1995. *The Imperative of Health: Public Health and the Regulated Body*. Sage Publications.

———. 1999. "Risk and the Ontology of Pregnant Embodiment." In *Risk and Sociocultural Theory: New Directions and Perspectives*, edited by D. Lupton. Cambridge University Press.

MacKendrick, Norah. 2018. *Better Safe Than Sorry: How Consumers Navigate Exposure to Everyday Toxics*. University of California Press.

Mahmood, Saba. 2001. "Feminist Theory, Embodiment, and the Docile Agent: Some Reflections on the Egyptian Islamic Revival." *Cultural Anthropology* 16(2):202–36.

———. 2012. *Politics of Piety: The Islamic Revival and the Feminist Subject*. Princeton University Press.

Malamud, Ofer, and Abigail Wozniak. 2010. *The Impact of College Education on Geographic Mobility: Identifying Education Using Multiple Components of Vietnam Draft Risk*. Working paper 16463. National Bureau of Economic Research. doi: 10.3386/w16463.

Mani, Anandi, Sendhil Mullainathan, Eldar Shafir, and Jiaying Zhao. 2013. "Poverty Impedes Cognitive Function." *Science* 341(6149):976–80. doi: 10.1126/science.1238041.

Marmot, Michael, and Richard Wilkinson. 2005. *Social Determinants of Health*. OUP Oxford.

Martin, Karin A. 1998. "Becoming a Gendered Body: Practices of Preschools." *American Sociological Review* 63(4):494–511. doi: 10.2307/2657264.

Mason, Katherine. 2012. "The Unequal Weight of Discrimination: Gender, Body Size, and Income Inequality." *Social Problems* 59(3):411–35. doi: 10.1525/sp.2012.59.3.411.

———. 2016a. "Responsible Bodies: Self-Care and State Power in the U.S. Women, Infants, and Children Program." *Social Politics: International Studies in Gender, State & Society* 23(1):70–93. doi: 10.1093/sp/jxv014.

———. 2016b. "Women, Infants, and (Fat) Children: Hidden 'Obesity Epidemic' Discourse and the Practical Politics of Health Promotion at WIC." *Fat Studies* 5(2):116–36. doi: 10.1080/21604851.2016.1144422.

Mayo Clinic. 2018. "Grocery Store Tour: Shopping the Perimeter." Mayo Clinic Health System, March 23. www.mayoclinichealthsystem.org.

McCormack, Karen. 2005. "Stratified Reproduction and Poor Women's Resistance." *Gender & Society* 19(5):660–79. doi: 10.1177/0891243205278010.

McMillan Cottom, Tressie. 2019. *Thick: and Other Essays.* New Press.

Mendes, Elizabeth. 2012. "Americans Spend $151 a Week on Food, the High-Income, $180." *Gallup*, August 2. www.gallup.com.

Messerschmidt, James W. 2011. "The Struggle for Heterofeminine Recognition: Bullying, Embodiment, and Reactive Sexual Offending by Adolescent Girls." *Feminist Criminology* 6(3):203–33. doi: 10.1177/1557085111408062.

Metzl, Jonathan. 2010. "Introduction: Why 'Against Health'?" Pp. 1–12 in *Against Health: How Health Became the New Morality*, edited by J. Metzl and A. Kirkland. NYU Press.

Momigliano, Anna. 2019. "Breast-Feeding Isn't Free: This Is How Much It Really Costs." *Washington Post*, May 21.

Monk, Ellis P., Michael H. Esposito, and Hedwig Lee. 2021. "Beholding Inequality: Race, Gender, and Returns to Physical Attractiveness in the United States." *American Journal of Sociology* 127(1):194–241. doi: 10.1086/715141.

Monsivais, Pablo, Anju Aggarwal, and Adam Drewnowski. 2014. "Time Spent on Home Food Preparation and Indicators of Healthy Eating." *American Journal of Preventive Medicine* 47(6):796–802. doi: 10.1016/j.amepre.2014.07.033.

Mooallem, Jon. 2018. "Once Prohibited, Women's Ski Jumping Is Set to Take Flight." *New York Times*, January 30.

Moore, Sarah E. H. 2010. "Is the Healthy Body Gendered? Toward a Feminist Critique of the New Paradigm of Health." *Body & Society* 16(2):95–118.

Moses, Marilyn C., and Roberto Hugh Potter. 2008. "The Use of Doulas for Inmates in Labor: Continuous Supportive Care with Positive Outcomes." *Corrections Today*, June 1:58–73.

Mude, William, Victor M. Oguoma, Tafadzwa Nyanhanda, Lillian Mwanri, and Carolyne Njue. 2021. "Racial Disparities in COVID-19 Pandemic Cases, Hospitalisations, and Deaths: A Systematic Review and Meta-Analysis." *Journal of Global Health* 11:05015. doi: 10.7189/jogh.11.05015.

Muñoz, José Esteban. 2013. *Disidentifications: Queers of Color and the Performance of Politics.* University of Minnesota Press.

Murkoff, Heidi, and Sharon Mazel. 2005. *What to Expect When You're Expecting.* 4th ed. Workman Publishing.

National Institutes of Health. 2018. "What Are the Benefits of Breastfeeding?" Eunice Kennedy Shriver National Institute of Child Health and Human Development, July 27. www.nichd.nih.gov.

Nelson, Margaret K. 1982. "The Effect of Childbirth Preparation on Women of Different Social Classes." *Journal of Health and Social Behavior* 23(4):339–52. doi: 10.2307/2136492.

Newman, Andrew Adam. 2012. "Marketing Wine as a Respite from Women's Many Roles." *New York Times*, August 30.

Nicholls, Emily. 2016. "'What on Earth Is She Drinking?': Doing Femininity through Drink Choice on the Girls' Night Out." *Journal of International Women's Studies* 17(2):77–91.

North, Anna. 2021. "How Emily Oster Became One of the Most Respected—and Reviled—Voices of the Pandemic." *Vox*, July 26. www.vox.com.

Oates, Gabriela R., Bradford E. Jackson, Edward E. Partridge, Karan P. Singh, Mona N. Fouad, and Sejong Bae. 2017. "Sociodemographic Patterns of Chronic Disease." *American Journal of Preventive Medicine* 52(1 Suppl 1):S31–39. doi: 10.1016/j.amepre.2016.09.004.

Oliveira, Victor, Elizabeth Racine, Jennifer Olmsted, and Linda M. Ghelfi. 2002. "The WIC Program: Background, Trends, and Issues." *Food Assistance and Nutrition Research Report* 27. US Department of Agriculture.

Oster, Emily. 2013. *Expecting Better: Why the Conventional Pregnancy Wisdom Is Wrong—and What You Really Need to Know*. Penguin.

Padilla-Walker, Laura M., Larry J. Nelson, and Jason S. Carroll. 2012. "Affording Emerging Adulthood: Parental Financial Assistance of Their College-Aged Children." *Journal of Adult Development* 19(1):50–58. doi: 10.1007/s10804-011 -9134-y.

Park, Julie J. 2019. "Inequality beyond Varsity Blues." *Contexts*, April 26. www.contexts.org.

Parsons, Talcott. 1951. "Illness and the Role of the Physician: A Sociological Perspective." *American Journal of Orthopsychiatry* 21(3):452–60. doi: 10.1111/j.1939-0025.1951.tb00003.x.

Pascoe, C. J. 2011. *Dude, You're a Fag: Masculinity and Sexuality in High School*. University of California Press.

Paul, Annie Murphy. 2010. "How the First Nine Months Shape the Rest of Your Life." *Time*, September 22.

Pearlstein, Joanna. 2019. "California's Vaccination Rate Slips as Medical Exemptions Rise." *Wired*, June 7. www.wired.com.

Pelters, Britta, and Barbro Wijma. 2016. "Neither a Sinner nor a Saint: Health as a Present-Day Religion in the Age of Healthism." *Social Theory & Health* 14(1):129–48. doi: 10.1057/sth.2015.21.

Penha-Lopes, Vânia. 2006. "'To Cook, Sew, to Be a Man': The Socialization for Competence and Black Men's Involvement in Housework." *Sex Roles* 54(3–4):261–74. doi: 10.1007/s11199-006-9343-1.

Peralta, Robert L. 2007. "College Alcohol Use and the Embodiment of Hegemonic Masculinity among European American Men." *Sex Roles* 56(11–12):741–56. doi: 10.1007/s11199-007-9233-1.

Petrzela, Natalia Mehlman. 2017. "Why Donald Trump's Diet Is Bad for America's Health." *Washington Post*, June 28.

Pew Research Center. 2015. "The American Family Today." Pew Research Center's Social & Demographic Trends Project, December 17. www.pewresearch.org.

Queen, Amazonian. 2016. "Biased, Poor Research." Customer review of *Expecting Better: Why the Conventional Pregnancy Wisdom Is Wrong—and What You Really Need to Know*, by Emily Oster. Amazon. Retrieved August 25, 2021. www.amazon.com.

Randles, Jennifer. 2021. "'Willing to Do Anything for My Kids': Inventive Mothering, Diapers, and the Inequalities of Carework." *American Sociological Review* 86(1):35–59. doi: 10.1177/0003122420977480.

Randles, Jennifer, and Kerry Woodward. 2018. "Learning to Labor, Love, and Live: Shaping the Good Neoliberal Citizen in State Work and Marriage Programs." *Sociological Perspectives* 61(1):39–56. doi: 10.1177/0731121417707753.

Reich, Jennifer A. 2012. *Fixing Families: Parents, Power, and the Child Welfare System*. Routledge.

———. 2016. *Calling the Shots: Why Parents Reject Vaccines*. NYU Press.

Riniolo, Todd C., Katherine C. Johnson, Tracy R. Sherman, and Julie A. Misso. 2006. "Hot or Not: Do Professors Perceived as Physically Attractive Receive Higher Student Evaluations?" *Journal of General Psychology* 133(1):19–35. doi: 10.3200/GENP.133.1.19–35.

Roberts, Dorothy. 1997. *Killing the Black Body: Race, Reproduction, and the Meaning of Liberty*. Vintage Books.

———. 2002. *Shattered Bonds: The Color of Child Welfare*. Basic Books.

Root, Maria P. R. 1991. "Persistent, Disordered Eating as a Gender-Specific, Post-Traumatic Stress Response to Sexual Assault." *Psychotherapy: Theory, Research, Practice, Training* 28(1):96–102. doi: 10.1037/0033–3204.28.1.96.

Ruiz, Juan Ignacio, Kaamel Nuhu, Justin Tyler McDaniel, Federico Popoff, Ariel Izcovich, and Juan Martin Criniti. 2015. "Inequality as a Powerful Predictor of Infant and Maternal Mortality around the World." *PLOS ONE* 10(10):e0140796. doi: 10.1371/journal.pone.0140796.

Saltonstall, Robin. 1993. "Healthy Bodies, Social Bodies: Men's and Women's Concepts and Practices of Health in Everyday Life." *Social Science & Medicine* 36(1):7–14. doi: 10.1016/0277–9536(93)90300-S.

Sayer, Liana C., and Leigh Fine. 2011. "Racial-Ethnic Differences in U.S. Married Women's and Men's Housework." *Social Indicators Research* 101(2):259–65. doi: 10.1007/s11205-010-9645-0.

Sears, Bill. 2020. "What Is Attachment Parenting?" Ask Dr Sears. www.askdrsears.com.

Senapathy, Kavin. 2016. "Yet Another Study Claims and Fails to Show That Breastfeeding Is Best." *Forbes*, December 20. www.forbes.com.

Shildrick, Margrit. 2015. *Leaky Bodies and Boundaries: Feminism, Postmodernism, and (Bio)Ethics*. Routledge.

Shilling, Chris. 1993. *The Body and Social Theory*. Sage Publications.

Siebers, Tobin. 2016. "Disability and the Theory of Complex Embodiment: For Identity Politics in a New Register." In *The Disability Studies Reader*, edited by L. J. Davis. Routledge.

Smith, Dorothy E. 1974. "Women's Perspective as a Radical Critique of Sociology." *Sociological Inquiry* 44(1):7–13. doi: 10.1111/j.1475-682X.1974.tb00718.x.

St. Louis, Brett. 2003. "Sport, Genetics, and the 'Natural Athlete': The Resurgence of Racial Science." *Body & Society* 9(2):75–95. doi: 10.1177/1357034X030092004.

Stalsberg, Ragna, and Arve Vorland Pedersen. 2018. "Are Differences in Physical Activity across Socioeconomic Groups Associated with Choice of Physical Activity Variables to Report?" *International Journal of Environmental Research and Public Health* 15(5):922. doi: 10.3390/ijerph15050922.

Stempel, Carl. 2005. "Adult Participation Sports as Cultural Capital: A Test of Bourdieu's Theory of the Field of Sports." *International Review for the Sociology of Sport* 40(4):411–32. doi: 10.1177/1012690206066170.

Strasser, Susan. 2000. *Never Done: A History of American Housework*. Macmillan.

Strings, Sabrina. 2019. *Fearing the Black Body: The Racial Origins of Fat Phobia*. NYU Press.

Tax Policy Center. 2020. "Household Income Quintiles." Tax Policy Center. Retrieved August 17, 2021. www.taxpolicycenter.org.

The Root Staff. 2014. "Why Do Black People Have So Many Cousins?" *Root*, July 30. www.theroot.com.

Thébaud, Sarah, Sabino Kornrich, and Leah Ruppanner. 2021. "Good Housekeeping, Great Expectations: Gender and Housework Norms." *Sociological Methods & Research* 50(3):1186–1214. doi: 10.1177/0049124119852395.

Tinsley, Omise'eke Natasha. 2018. *Ezili's Mirrors: Imagining Black Queer Genders*. Duke University Press.

Topol, Eric J., Abraham Verghese, and Katelyn K. Jetelina. 2022. "COVID Vaccines for the Under 5's: The 'Finish Line' We Need." *Medscape*, February 17. www.medscape.com.

US Department of Agriculture (USDA) Economic Research Service. 2011. "Annual State Agricultural Exports Interactive Chart." Economic Research Service. www.ers.usda.gov.

US Department of Health & Human Services. 2021. "Sexual Assault." Office on Women's Health, February 15. www.womenshealth.gov.

Villarosa, Linda. 2018. "Why America's Black Mothers and Babies Are in a Life-or-Death Crisis." *New York Times*, April 11.

Waggoner, Miranda R. 2015. "Cultivating the Maternal Future: Public Health and the Prepregnant Self." *Signs: Journal of Women in Culture and Society* 40(4):939–62. doi: 10.1086/680404.

———. 2017. *The Zero Trimester: Pre-Pregnancy Care and the Politics of Reproductive Risk*. University of California Press.

Washington, Harriet A. 2008. *Medical Apartheid: The Dark History of Medical Experimentation on Black Americans from Colonial Times to the Present*. Knopf Doubleday.

Waytz, Adam, Kelly M. Hoffman, and Sophie Trawalter. 2012. "Racial Bias in Perceptions of Others' Pain." *PLOS ONE* 7(11):e48546. doi: 10.1371/journal.pone.0048546.

West, Candace, and Don H. Zimmerman. 1987. "Doing Gender." *Gender & Society* 1(2):125–51.

Westwood, Ryan. 2018. "5 Reasons Why Sporting a Staff of Athletes Is a Game-Winning Strategy." *Forbes*, May 19. www.forbes.com.

Wilkinson, Richard, and Kate Pickett. 2011. *The Spirit Level: Why Greater Equality Makes Societies Stronger*. Bloomsbury Publishing USA.

Williams, Clare. 2000. "Doing Health, Doing Gender: Teenagers, Diabetes, and Asthma." *Social Science & Medicine* 50(3):387–96. doi: 10.1016/S0277-9536(99)00340-8.

Williams, David R. 2012. "Miles to Go before We Sleep: Racial Inequities in Health." *Journal of Health and Social Behavior* 53(3):279–95. doi: 10.1177/0022146512455804.

Williams, Janet F., Vincent C. Smith, and the Committee on Substance Abuse. 2015. "Fetal Alcohol Spectrum Disorders." *Pediatrics* 136(5):e1395–1406. doi: 10.1542/peds.2015-3113.

Willis, Paul. 2017. *Learning to Labour: How Working-Class Kids Get Working-Class Jobs*. Routledge.

Wolf, Naomi. 2003. *Misconceptions: Truth, Lies, and the Unexpected on the Journey to Motherhood*. Anchor Books.

Wright, Erik Olin, Karen Shire, Shu-Ling Hwang, Maureen Dolan, and Janeen Baxter. 1992. "The Non-Effects of Class on the Gender Division of Labor in the Home: A Comparative Study of Sweden and the United States." *Gender & Society* 6(2):252–82. doi: 10.1177/089124392006002008.

Wu, Lei Lei. 2021. "Vaccine 'Belief Exemption' Bans No Panacea for Stopping Measles Outbreaks." *Medpage Today*, December 7. Retrieved February 26, 2022. www.medpagetoday.com.

Young, Iris Marion. 1990. *Throwing like a Girl and Other Essays in Feminist Philosophy and Social Theory*. Indiana University Press.

Zelizer, Viviana A. 1994. *Pricing the Priceless Child*. Princeton University Press.

Zipprich, Jennifer, Kathleen Winter, Jill Hacker, Dongxiang Xia, James Watt, and Kathleen Harriman. 2015. "Measles Outbreak: California, December 2014–February 2015." *Morbidity and Mortality Weekly Report* 64(06):153–54.

Zola, Irving Kenneth. 1972. "Medicine as an Institution of Social Control." *Sociological Review* 20(4):487–504. doi: 10.1111/j.1467-954X.1972.tb00220.x.

# INDEX

AAP. *See* American Academy of Pediatrics

achieved status, 7, 10, 12, 33–34, 217, 226

ACOG. *See* American College of Obstetricians and Gynecologists

Acosta, Rosa (LL group), 46–47

adversity, agency response to, 189, 191; HH and, 180–84; LL and, 184; maternal embodiment flexibility for, 184–88; rigidity and flexibility for, 182–84

advice. *See* grandmother advice; health professionals and expert advice; peer advice; physician advice

agency, 161–62, 191; adversity response and, 180–89; bodily sensations during pregnancy and, 169; challenges to, 168–71; control cultivation and, 163–66; Denbow on, 170–71, 179; embodiment of, 163–71; Mahmood on, 170, 171; in risk-assessing paradigm, 112; self-control and social status for, 166–68; structural limitations acknowledgement and, 177–79. *See also* flexible agency response, of LL; rigid agency response, of HH

alcohol consumption, 251n4; AAP on, 117; CDC on, 117–18; cessation of, 105; HH participants on, 118–19, 129, 251n24; wine cultural connotation for, 118–19, 122–23

alternative identification, among LL, 150–57

ambivalence, over grandmother advice, 48, 51–52

American Academy of Allergy, Asthma, and Immunology, on three-day wait rule feeding plan, 76

American Academy of Pediatrics (AAP): on alcohol consumption, 117; breast is best recommendation of, 2, 41, 104, 145, 176; on rice cereal addition for GERD, 120–21

American College of Obstetricians and Gynecologists (ACOG): on exercise in pregnancy, 133, 252n8; on pregnancy monitoring, 85–86

anorexia, 51, 80–83, 87–88, 98

anticipatory motherhood, of Waggoner, 88–89, 92, 123, 130

ascribed status, 7, 10, 226

Asian and Latina immigrant identities, 150–52

AskMoxie.com, 41

aspirational identities, of LL women, 60–61, 66, 155–57, 220

athleticism: HH on self-identity and, 131–34, 218; Stemple on professional success and, 217

attachment parenting, 63, 116, 165, 251n2, 251n20, 252n3

*Baby Book* (Sears), 42

Babycenter.com, 41, 103

Baker, Becky (LL group): birth plan lack by, 185; negative breastfeeding experience of, 62; on peer support, 62–63

Barber, Kristen, 217

bed sharing, 250n10, 255n4; breastfeeding and, 108; risk-assessing on, 108, 117

Begovic, Masha (HH group): child vaccination resistance of, 56–57; rigid agency and pregnancy goals of, 172–73

middle- and upper-class women (*cont.*)
medical and scientific knowledge
role for, 40, 230; medical authority
challenge from, 43; midwife or doulas
childbirth choice of, 44; moderation,
cosmopolitanism, informed consumption values of, 198–202, 212; mommy
groups for peer advice response
from, 53–59, 103; PBEs and, 56; peer
advice response for, 53–57, 219; peers
and, 53–57, 61, 64, 138–40; physician
advice response of, 40–45; physicians
challenge from, 42–44, 123; Reich on
child vaccination skepticism of, 57;
reproductive body projects connection
with self-identity of, 25; risk-avoidant
paradigm and, 5, 24, 98–103, 123; self-
control and social status of, 166–68;
self-identity and, 126, 128–37, 148, 223;
social status and, 79, 166–68; taste of
luxury of, 9, 226; teaching children as
informed consumers by, 194, 200–201.
*See also* rigid agency response, of HH;
*specific HH participants*
midwife, 255n11; HH childbirth choice of,
44; LL women and, 189; water birth
delivery and, 185–86
mixed-class group (low-education, high-
income) (LH) and (high-education,
low-income) (HL): body-care practices link to social status, 223; on breastfeeding, 210, 221–22; characteristics of,
21; children classy bodies cultivation
by, 210–13; on choices and class implications, 20, 160; cultural or material
forces in class differences of, 19–20;
education level influence on, 220–21;
financial freedom or constraint of,
220–21; health literacy and information gathering by, 220–22; ideological
differences in bodily distinction of,
220, 222–23; mommy groups for peer
advice participation of, 55, 58–59, 65;

no cost is too great mindset and, 115–
16; religious identities of, 152–55; WIC
good but simple description by, 38–39,
64, 206, 222. *See also specific LH or HL
participants*
moderation: health and body-care
practices extremes and, 138–40; as HH
value, 198–202, 212
mommy groups, for peer advice, 141–42;
HH response to, 53–59, 103; HL and
LH participation in, 55, 58–59, 65;
horizontal relationship in, 57; LL
participation in, 58–64, 66
moral good, health as stratified, 10–12,
159–60
moral judgment, risk-avoidant paradigm
and, 97, 122
Moran, Charlotte (HH group): on alcohol
consumption, 119; caffeine cessation
of, 105; on husband and health- and
development-related decisions, 74;
on peer advice trust, 53; on physician
advice and alternative sources, 40–41;
rigid agency and postpartum goals of,
173, 191; whole foods preference of, 129
Mormon religious identity, 152
motherhood: bodily demands of, 4;
Dow on Black people good values of
motherhood, 176–77; Dow on integrative, 177; scientific, 99, 111; Waggoner
anticipatory, 88–89, 92, 123, 130
mothering advice magazines, 102
mothering websites, for peer advice, 54–
55, 58, 65
Muñoz, José Esteban, 147

National Institutes of Health (NIH),
breastfeeding recommendation of, 104
natural childbirth, 182–84, 232; athletic
identity and, 132; Gaskin on intense
labor in, 22
natural growth practices, Lareau on, 197
Nelson, Margaret K., 185

NIH. *See* National Institutes of Health

Noble, Lara (HH group): on information gathering to provide to husband, 74–75; pre-pregnancy eating disorder of, 80, 231–32; self-identity narrative and unhealthful behaviors of, 129–30

no cost is too great mindset, of risk-avoidant paradigm, 5, 24, 99, 108, 113, 115–16

normalizing judgment, 31–33

noticing, of children body-care needs: gendered division in, 68–72, 94–95; women explanation for, 70–71

Novak, Anya (HH group), on children moderation, 201–2

nuclear family, idealization of, 63

nutrition: children strategies of WIC, 3, 36–37, 205–6; eating disorder and knowledge of, 80–83, 96; education for fathers by WIC, 93–94; food choices and, 92–93, 125, 126, 150–51; LL assistance through WIC, 35; primal eating and, 125–26, 252n3. *See also* diets; feeding plans; foods; healthy eating

Oates, Gabriela, 254n10

O'Brien, Lynne (LL group): on children ill health aversion, 207–8; gestational diabetes of, 208; personal failure frame of, 142–43; WIC positive experiences of, 35–36

Oster, Emily, 109–10

out of control feelings, of maternal body, 25, 180–81

Park, Ji-Eun (HL group), 151; birth plan lack of, 185

Pascoe, C. J., 216

Paul, Annie Murphy, 91

PBEs. *See* personal belief exemptions

*Pediatrics* (journal), 42

peer advice: HH response to, 53–59, 103; LL response to, 58–64, 66; mommy groups for, 53–66, 103, 141–42; Moran HH on trust of, 53; mothering websites for, 54–55, 58, 65; from older person, 60; risk-avoidant paradigm and, 53; unhelpful, harmful health from, 55–57; vertical element of, 59

peers: HH and, 53–57, 61, 64, 138–40; identity and selection of, 53–55, 61; LL and, 58–64, 66; moderation and extremes of, 138–40; support of, 62–63

Peralta, Louise (LH group): bodily vulnerability and rape of, 82; on mothering website social exclusion, 54–55, 58, 65

personal belief exemptions (PBEs), for vaccinations, 56

personal failure frames, of LL disidentification, 142–44

personal taste frames, of LL disidentification, 144–47, 160

Peters, Kimberly (HH group), 165–66

physician advice: alternative sources to, 40–41; HH challenge to, 42–44, 123; HH response to, 40–45; for postpartum women, 34; relationship and, 39–40

Pollan, Michael, 193

poor and working-class women (low-education, low-income) (LL), 5, 19, 26, 234; agency response to adversity by, 184; alternative identification among, 150–57; aspirational identities of, 60–61, 66, 155–57, 220; birth plan lack of strong preferences of, 186–88; on breastfeeding, 113–14, 143–46, 175–76, 222; characteristics of, 20–21; children social inequality and, 204; class cultural differences and, 100; cleanliness, clear rules and health priorities of, 202–10; fear of food waste by, 224, 254n2; financial and material resources constraints for, 100; grandmother advice and, 45–49; health and body-care practices response of, 219, 223–24;

# ABOUT THE AUTHOR

KATHERINE MASON is Assistant Professor of Sociology and Women's & Gender Studies at Wheaton College in Massachusetts. A paper based on this project won the Graduate Student Best Paper Award from the American Sociological Association's Section on Body and Embodiment. She is coeditor, with Natalie Boero, of *The Oxford Handbook of the Sociology of Body and Embodiment.*